Saintly Men of Nursing

Saintly Men of Nursing
100 AMAZING STORIES

Fr. Robert J. Kus

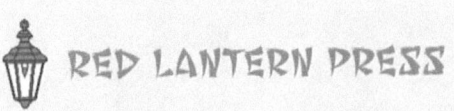

Wilmington, North Carolina

www.redlanternpress.com

© 2017 Fr. Robert J. Kus
All rights reserved.

ISBN: 1548685364
ISBN 9781548685362

The Cover

THE FRONT COVER OF THIS book, a painting done by artist Alessandro Giambra, shows six of the 100 saintly men of nursing whose stories grace these pages. The six men are, from top left and going in a clockwise direction: Venerable Nicola D'Onofrio, St. Martin de Porres, St. Francis of Assisi, St. Camillus de Lellis, St. John of God, and St. Damien of Molokai.

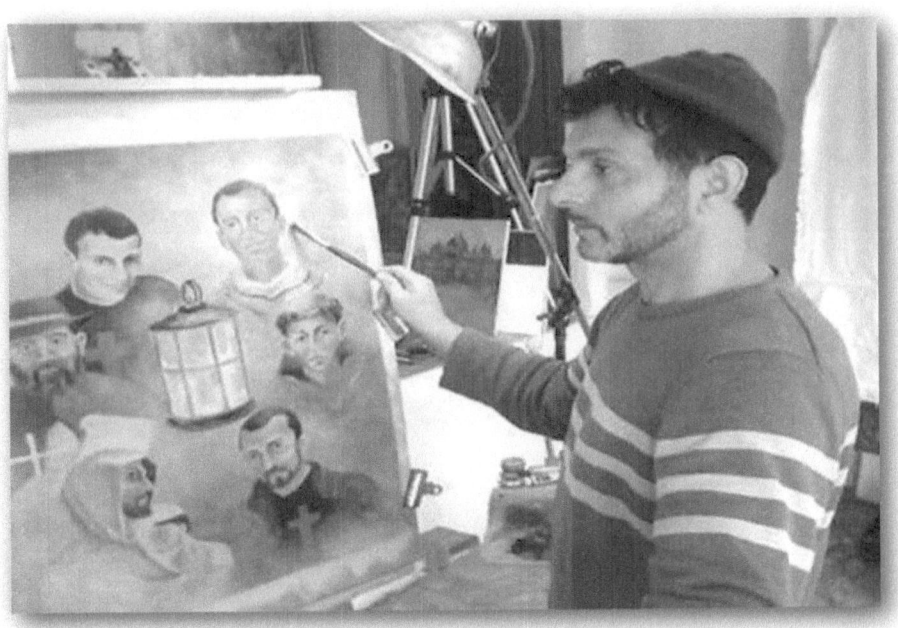

Alessandro Giambra, originally from Italy, teaches Italian, art theory and painting in the St. Mary Adult School on the campus of the Basilica Shrine of St. Mary, Wilmington, North Carolina.

Publications of Red Lantern Press

Journals by Fr. Robert J. Kus

- Dreams for the Vineyard: Journal of a Parish Priest - 2002
- For Where Your Treasure Is: Journal of a Parish Priest – 2003
- There Will Your Heart Be Also: Journal of a Parish Priest – 2004
- Field of Plenty: Journal of a Parish Priest – 2005
- Called to the Coast: Journal of a Parish Priest – 2006
- Then Along Came Marcelino: Journal of a Parish Priest – 2007
- Living the Dream: Journal of a Parish Priest – 2008
- A Hand to Honduras: Journal of a Parish Priest – 2009
- Beacon of Hope: Journal of a Parish Priest – 2010
- Serving God By Serving Others: Journal of a Parish Priest – 2011
- The Year of Clifton: Journal of a Parish Priest – 2012
- Basilica: Journal of a Parish Priest – 2013
- Crucifix: Journal of a Parish Priest – 2014
- Holy Doors: Journal of a Parish Priest – 2015

Homily Collections by Fr. Robert J. Kus

- Flowers in the Wind 1 – Story-Based Homilies for Cycle B
- Flowers in the Wind 2 – Story-Based Homilies for Cycle C
- Flowers in the Wind 3 – Story-Based Homilies for Cycle A
- Flowers in the Wind 4 – More Story-Based Homilies for Cycle A
- Flowers in the Wind 5 – More Story-Based Homilies for Cycle B
- Flowers in the Wind 6 – More Story-Based Homilies for Cycle C
- Flowers in the Wind 7 – Still More Story-Based Homilies for Cycle A

Nursing and Saints by Fr. Robert J. Kus

- Saintly Men of Nursing: 100 Amazing Stories

Dedication

To all men of nursing –

Past, Present, and Future

Acknowledgments

MANY THANKS GO TO ALL the nurses I have known and served with throughout the years throughout the United States. They have enriched my life in many ways.

Thanks go to Pat Marriott who edited this book, and to Alessandro Giambra who painted the cover for the book.

Special thanks also go to the fine folks of CreateSpace who helped bring this book to life.

Table of Contents

Introduction · xvii

1	St. Aimo, O.S.B. ·	1
2	Fr. Alonso de Sandoval, S.J. ·	3
3	St. Aloysius Gonzaga, S.J. ·	5
4	Ven. Andrew Beltrami, S.D.B. · · · · · · · · · · · · · · · · · · ·	9
5	St. André Bessette, C.S.C. ·	11
6	St. Anthelm of Belley, O.Cart. · · · · · · · · · · · · · · · · · · ·	13
7	Bl. Anthony Manzi ·	15
8	St. Anthony Mary Pucci, O.S.M. · · · · · · · · · · · · · · · · · ·	17
9	Bl. Arnold Reche, F.S.C. ·	19
10	St. Benedict of Nursia, O.S.B. · · · · · · · · · · · · · · · · · · ·	21
11	St. Benedict Menni, O.H. ·	23
12	Bl. Benito Solana Ruiz, C.P. ·	27
13	Bl. Bentivoglio de Bonis, O.F.M. · · · · · · · · · · · · · · · · · ·	29
14	Bl. Benvenuto of Gubbio, O.F.M. · · · · · · · · · · · · · · · · · ·	31
15	Bro. Bernardino de Obregón, O.M. · · · · · · · · · · · · · · · · ·	33
16	St. Bernardino of Siena, O.F.M. · · · · · · · · · · · · · · · · · · ·	35
17	St. Bernard of Corleone, O.F.M. Cap. · · · · · · · · · · · · · · ·	37
18	St. Bernardo Tolomei, O.S.B. Oliv. · · · · · · · · · · · · · · · · ·	41
19	St. Cajetan, C.R. ·	43
20	St. Camillus de Lellis, M.I. ·	45
21	St. Carthach (Mo Chutu) of Lismore · · · · · · · · · · · · · · · ·	47

22	St. Charles of Sezze, O.F.M.	49
23	St. Crispin of Viterbo, O.F.M. Cap	51
24	St. Damien of Molokai, SS.CC.	53
25	St. Didacus (Diego), O.F.M.	57
26	Bl. Edward J.M. Poppe	59
27	Bl. Engelmar Unzeitig, C.M.M.	61
28	Bl. Enrico Rebuchini, M.I.	63
29	St. Fidelis of Sigmaringen, O.F.M. Cap.	65
30	St. Finnian of Clonard	67
31	St. Francis of Assisi, O.F.M.	69
32	St. Francis Mary of Camporosso, O.F.M. Cap.	71
33	St. Francis Xavier, S.J.	73
34	Bl. Francis Xavier Seelos, C.Ss.R.	77
35	St. Gaspar Bertoni, C.S.S.	81
36	St. Gerard Majella, C.Ss.R.	83
37	Bl. Gerard Meccati	87
38	Bl. Gerard Thom	89
39	St. Gerlac	91
40	St. Henry Morse, S.J.	93
41	Fr. Henri Nouwen	95
42	Bl. Hugolino of Magalotti, O.S.F.	99
43	St. Ivo of Brittany	101
44	Bl. James of Bitetto, O.F.M.	103
45	Bl. James of Lodi, O.S.F.	105
46	Bl. Jeremy of Valacchia, O.F.M. Cap.	107
47	St. Jerome Emiliani, C.R.S.	109
48	St. John Baptist de Rossi	111
49	St. John Bosco, S.D.B.	113
50	St. John Calabria, P.S.D.P.	117
51	Bl. John Colombini	119
52	St. John of the Cross, O.C.D.	121
53	St. John Eudes, C.J.M.	123
54	St. John of God, O.H.	125

55	St. John Grande-Román, O.H.	127
56	St. John Leonardi, O.M.D.	129
57	Bl. John Pelingotto, O.S.F.	131
58	St. José Gabriel del Rosario Brochero, T.O.S.D.	133
59	Bl. José Tarrats Comaposada, S.J.	135
60	St. Joseph Benedict Cottolengo	137
61	St. Joseph Calasanz, Sch.P.	141
62	Bro. Joseph Dutton	145
63	St. Joseph Freinademetz, S.V.D.	149
64	Bl. Joseph Gerard, O.M.I.	153
65	St. Joseph Oriol	155
66	Bl. Juan Agustín Codera-Marqués, S.D.B.	159
67	Bl. Juan Bautista Egozcuezábal-Aldaz, O.H.	161
68	St. Juan Macías, O.P.	163
69	Bro. Juan de Mena, O.P.	165
70	St. Justin de Jacobis, C.M.	167
71	Bl. Liberatus Weiss, O.F.M.	169
72	Bl. Luchesio Modestini, O.F.S.	171
73	St. Louis Bertrán, O.P.	173
74	St. Ludovico of Casoria, O.F.M.	175
75	Bl. Luigi Maria Monti, C.F.I.C.	177
76	Bl. Luke Belludi, O.F.M.	179
77	St. Martin de Porres, O.P.	181
78	Bl. Michael Pius Fasoli, O.F.M.	185
79	St. Michael Kozaki, O.F.S.	187
80	Bl. Michael Rua, S.D.B.	189
81	Ven. Nicola D'Onofrio, M.I.	191
82	Bl. Oddino Barrotti, O.S.F.	195
83	St. Paul of the Cross, C.P.	197
84	St. Peter of St. Joseph de Betancur, O.F.B.	199
85	St. Peter Claver, S.J.	203
86	Bl. Peter Donders, C.Ss.R.	207
87	Bl. Peter Tecelano, O.F.S.	209

88	St. Philip Neri, C.O.	211
89	Bl. Pier Giorgio Frassati, T.O.S.D.	213
90	Bl. Raphael Chylinski, O.F.M. Conv.	217
91	Bl. Raymond of Capua, O.P.	219
92	St. Rock	221
93	St. Salvius of Albi, O.S.B.	223
94	Bl. Samuel Marzorati, O.F.M.	225
95	St. Simon of Lipnicza, O.F.M.	227
96	Ven. Simon Srugi, S.D.B.	229
97	Bl. Stephen Bellesini, O.S.A.	231
98	St. Toribio Romo-González	233
99	Bl. Vivaldo Stricchi, O.S.F.	237
100	St. Zygmunt Gorazdowski	239
	Selected Bibliography	241

Introduction

THE PURPOSE OF THIS BOOK is to introduce the reader to 100 saintly men who, at least some times in their lives, were nurses. I wrote this book in honor of my 50th anniversary as an R.N.

All of the men in this book were Catholic Christians, but I'm sure that there are many other men who did nursing and led holy lives. Their stories are for another author to tell.

Some of the men did nursing for just small parts of their lives, such as those who nursed in epidemics that came to their towns. Others dedicated their lives to nursing, such St. John of God and St. Camillus de Lellis.

These 100 saintly men of nursing are most likely just the "tip of the iceberg," for it is probable that most saintly men of nursing will never be identified as such. Some men, for example, were martyred in groups. Their martyrdom made them famous, not their nursing. For example, 71 Hospitaller martyrs were beatified in 1992. Because many of the men of the Hospitaller Order are nurses, many of these martyrs were undoubtedly nurses. And, of course, some saintly men of nursing will never be identified for their nursing because their stories or their nursing activities were not recorded.

Many of the men in this book have more than one name – names given them by their parents, and names they took when they joined religious orders. Thus, for example, St. John of the Cross's name before entering religious life was Juan de Yepes y Álvarez. The names used in the text are the ones by which they are best known.

Though this book should prove especially interesting to men of nursing and nursing historians, I think that anyone who is interested in seeing how saintly people live their lives to make the world a better place will be very pleased to meet these 100 men.

Enjoy and be inspired!

Fr. Robert J. Kus
Basilica Shrine of St. Mary
Wilmington, N.C.
August 2017

1

St. Aimo, O.S.B.
d. 1173

Aimo was born near Rennes, France. As a young man, he became a Benedictine monk in what today is Normandy.

In his monastery, he was responsible for nursing two monks of the community who were suffering from leprosy.

Brother Aimo served these two men not only with great compassion, but without fear. Many of the other monks of the community came to the conclusion that perhaps Aimo himself had leprosy. Therefore, Aimo served as a lay brother.

When it became obvious that Aimo did not have the disease, the superiors of the monastery chose him to be ordained to the priesthood.

In addition to his compassionate nursing practice, Fr. Aimo was noted for having mystical experiences during his life.

St. Aimo's feast day is April 30.

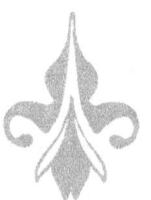

2

Fr. Alonso de Sandoval, S.J.
December 7, 1576 – December 25, 1652

ALONSO DE SANDOVAL WAS BORN on December 7, 1576 in Seville. His family moved to Peru around 1583 or 1584.

When he grew up, Alonso entered the Society of Jesus (Jesuits) in 1593. At the time he lived, the Jesuit seminary in Lima was an excellent educational institution. The Jesuits there had a wonderful library and had one of the first printing presses in that part of the world. They also encouraged their men to be writers.

Fr. Alonso was assigned to Cartagena, now part of Colombia. There he found the African slave trade in full force. With a clear vision and incredible passion, Fr. Alonso did all he could for the slaves. He nursed them whenever he could in mind, body and spirit. He nursed their multiple health problems: yellow fever, smallpox, terror, suicidal ideation, and a host of other health problems. Moreover, he taught them the faith. He also fought a losing battle in a quest to have slaves treated humanely.

Fr. Alonso was not only a priest and a nurse. He also used ethnographic research methods of what would come to be called sociology and cultural anthropology, to document the African slaves' lives and culture. He was probably the greatest ethnographer of the African slave experience in all of South America.

Father Alonso faithfully served the slaves of Cartagena for 45 years. In 1651 an epidemic of some sort swept across the area, and Fr. Alonso became ill.

After two years confined to bed, Fr. Alonso de Sandoval died on Christmas Day, 1652.

Fortunately, another priest would come to take his place to nurse the sick and provide for their spiritual care, St. Peter Claver (another Saintly Man of Nursing in this book).

3

St. Aloysius Gonzaga, S.J.
March 9, 1568 – June 21, 1591

Aloysius Gonzaga was born on March 9, 1568 in his family's castle in Castiglione, Italy. His father was the eldest son of the Marquis of Castiglione, and his mother was the daughter of a baron.

Because his father wanted him to become a soldier, he sent little Aloysius to a military camp when Aloysius was only five years old. Though this delighted Aloysius' father, it made his mother angry because of the vulgar and blasphemous language the little boy picked up from the soldiers.

When Aloysius was growing up, there was much violence among men, and he witnessed the killing of two of his brothers.

When he was eight years old, Aloysius and his brother Rodolf were sent to Florence to receive their educations. In Florence, Aloysius developed a kidney disease that would remain with him for the rest of his life. While in Florence, Aloysius fell in love with reading the lives of the saints. He also developed a strong prayer life.

In July of 1580, Cardinal Charles Borromeo, who would one day be canonized, gave Aloysius First Communion. During this time, Aloysius continued reading about saints. It was after reading the lives of Jesuit missionary priests in India that Aloysius decided to follow a priestly calling.

To practice for his future life, Aloysius began to teach catechism to young boys in the summer months, and he adopted an ascetic life.

After serving for a brief time at a royal court in Spain, Aloysius announced his desire to enter the Society of Jesus (Jesuits) to study for the priesthood. Though his mother approved, Aloysius' father was very much opposed. Aloysius, however, had a very strong will; once he made up his mind about something, he was not easily dissuaded. When Aloysius' father could not get him to change his mind about being a priest, he tried to get Aloysius to be a diocesan priest instead of a Jesuit. His pleas fell on deaf ears: Aloysius entered the Society of Jesus in November of 1585 and gave up all right to his inheritance.

On November 25, 1585, Aloysius became a Jesuit novice in Rome. There his superiors told him that he must modify his severe lifestyle and become more social with other seminarians. In other words, he was told he had to "lighten up" for spiritual growth or he would burn himself out in no time.

During his novitiate, Aloysius experienced frequent headaches, kidney problems, skin disease, and insomnia. After his novitiate, the Jesuits sent him to Milan to study, but because of his poor health, he was sent back to Rome.

On November 25, 1587, Aloysius took vows of poverty, chastity, and obedience, and in March of 1588, he began his theology studies.

In 1589, an epidemic of the plague broke out in Rome, and the Jesuits opened a hospital for plague victims. Aloysius promptly volunteered to do nursing there. His supervisors agreed to let him practice nursing in the hospital, but because they did not want to lose him, they insisted that he serve only on nursing units that had no plague victims.

Not only did Aloysius prove to be an effective nurse, he also walked the streets of Rome, begging for alms for the patients' care.

Unbeknown to Aloysius or his superiors, there was a man already infected in the ward to which he was assigned. Soon, Aloysius showed signs of the plague and was anointed in preparation for his death.

Everyone was shocked, however, when Aloysius recovered. Unfortunately, however, his health became worse than ever.

In 1590, Aloysius had a vision from the Archangel Gabriel telling him that he would die within a year. Aloysius told everyone he would die during the Octave of the Feast of Corpus Christi.

Aloysius, after receiving the Sacrament of the Sick from Cardinal Bellarmine, died on June 21, 1591.

Pope Paul V canonized him on December 31, 1726.

St. Aloysius' feast day is June 21. He is a patron saint of youth.

4

Ven. Andrew Beltrami, S.D.B.
June 24, 1870 – December 30, 1897

ANDREW BELTRAMI WAS BORN ON June 24, 1870 in Omegna, Italy.

In October 1883, his parents sent him to the Salesian College at Lanzo. While there, he discerned that God was calling him to become a member of the Salesian Order. His mother told the novice master, "Make him a saint."

In 1886, the Salesian founder, Fr. John Bosco, gave Andrew his Salesian habit. Following his novitiate, Andrew completed two three-year courses of study successfully, showing his facility for academics.

As a young Salesian, Fr. Andrew got to know a Polish prince by the name of Augustus Czartoyski. The two quickly became very close friends. So when Augustus became ill with tuberculosis, it was Andrew who nursed him. In looking back on this nursing experience, Andrew wrote, "I am aware that I have been looking after a saint, an angel."

Fr. Andrew also became sick, but that did not slow him down. On the contrary, he threw himself into contemplation and writing. Specifically, he wrote about the works of St. Francis de Sales.

Fr. Andrew died on December 30, 1897 at the age of 27. He was buried in his hometown of Omegna.

Pope Paul VI declared Andrew to be a Venerable on December 5, 1966.

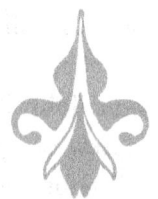

5
St. André Bessette, C.S.C.
August 9, 1845 – January 6, 1937

ALFRED BESSETTE WAS BORN ON August 9, 1845 in Mont-Saint-Grégoire, Quebec, the eighth of twelve children.

Because he was a frail infant, his parents had him baptized when he was only one day old.

Alfred's father was a carpenter and lumberman, and his mother was a homemaker who homeschooled the children.

When he was 12 years old, Alfred was orphaned and had to work for his living, taking many jobs including blacksmith, shoemaker, farmhand, and factory worker in the United States during the Civil War.

Experiencing a call to Religious life when he was 25 years old, Alfred joined the Congregation of the Holy Cross. After his novitiate, however, the Order would not accept Alfred because of his weak health. A bishop, however, intervened on his behalf, and the Congregation took him in as a Brother.

In Religious life, Alfred took the name André and became the porter, or doorkeeper, at Notre Dame College in Cote-des-Neiges, Quebec. He also worked as a sacristan, laundry worker, and messenger.

Brother André had a great love for St. Joseph, and that love is something for which he is noted. In fact, Brother André decided to build a church for St. Joseph on Mount Royal, and in 1904 he began raising money for the project.

As time went on, people began noticing that Brother André had a special love of the sick. He used to rub blessed oil on those who came to him with problems; this he named "St. Joseph's oil." Many people were cured and attributed their cure to Brother André and the oil. Brother André, however, realized he was a mere instrument of God and not a "miracle worker."

When an epidemic broke out in a nearby college, Brother André volunteered to work as a nurse. Not one of his patients died. Soon many sick people began to seek him out.

As his reputation began to soar, others began to pay closer attention to André. His superiors in the Congregation didn't know what to make of all the cures. Medical professionals became jealous and suspicious of Brother André, and many physicians began calling him a quack.

Nevertheless, because of his amazing success as a nurse, his superiors gave him four secretaries to handle the 80,000 letters he received each year. His assistance to people via letters was evidence of Brother André's skill in psychosocial nursing. Eventually, his superiors even gave him permission to visit the sick in a train station because the College was not able to handle the hordes of people flocking to him on their campus.

In 1924, the Congregation began to build Brother André's dream church – the Oratory of St. Joseph. In 1931, when the money ran out, Brother André directed the workers, "Put a statue of St. Joseph in the middle. If he wants a roof over his head, he'll get it." Needless to say, the church was built, and today it is a major pilgrimage site for people from all over the world.

On January 6, 1937, Brother André died at the age of 91. This age is remarkable considering that his Order almost didn't accept him because of his fragile health. Over 1,000,000 people filed past his coffin. In a sense, the people had already proclaimed him a saint at his death.

Pope Benedict XVI canonized him on October 17, 2010.

St. André's feast day is January 6.

6

St. Anthelm of Belley, O.Cart.
1107 - June 26, 1178

ANTHELM WAS BORN IN 1107 in a castle in Savoy.

When he grew up, he became a priest. However, when he was thirty years old, he left the parish priesthood to become a Carthusian monk at Portes. The Carthusian Order is one of the strictest religious communities in the Catholic Church. In fact, Carthusians often say that their Order has "never been reformed because it was never deformed."

In just two years, Anthelm became the Prior of the Order's motherhouse, Grand Chartreuse. In this position, he proved to be a wonderful administrator. Soon, the Order grew in numbers and in devotion. In Anthelm's administration, he improved buildings, built an aqueduct, and built a defensive wall. The rules of the Order were standardized, and women were allowed to become Carthusian nuns. Further, Anthelm brought other houses of the Order closer together.

Fr. Anthelm served in administration of his Order for 24 years, except for a few years when he lived as a hermit. In addition to helping his Order, he also defended Pope Alexander III against the antipope Victor IV. For his service, Pope Alexander III made Anthelm the Bishop of Belley in 1163. As bishop, Anthelm worked to bring order to his diocese and reform the clergy, many of whom had become lax in their priesthood.

Although Pope Alexander III deputized Bishop Anthelm to go to England to see if he could reconcile King Henry II and Thomas Becket, his poor health made a trip to England impossible. Instead, Anthelm returned to Belley, where he devoted his time to nursing lepers of the area and caring for the poor.

Bishop Anthelm died in Belley on June 26, 1178. His feast day is June 26. In religious art, St. Anthelm is portrayed holding a lamp lit by a divine hand.

7

Bl. Anthony Manzi
1237 - 1267

ANTHONY MANZI – ALSO KNOWN as Anthony Manzoni or "Anthony the Pilgrim" – was born in Padua sometime in 1237. His family was wealthy, and they were very religious Catholic Christians.

When his father died, and after Anthony was old enough to take charge of the family's riches, Anthony gave away the family fortune to the poor. This action enraged his two sisters, because it meant they would not have wedding dowries. Anthony's action also angered his townspeople, because they could not understand why he would give up his station in life to enter into a lower one.

Rejected by the people of Padua, Anthony left the town dressed as a pilgrim and eventually settled in Bazano, near Bologna. It was in Bazano that he began his nursing career. For three years, Anthony did private duty nursing for an elderly priest. For these three years, Anthony not only nursed the priest, but he would wander the streets begging for food, money, and other supplies to support his patient and himself.

When his priest-patient died, Anthony decided to become a religious pilgrim, visiting the popular Catholic pilgrimage sites of Europe – Rome, Loreto, Compostela, Cologne, and Jerusalem.

After much travel to these European destinations, Anthony returned to his hometown of Padua. There he found the people, including his two sisters who were now Religious Sisters, still hated him. So, he lived in the colonnade of a church outside the walls of the city. There, he soon died in 1267.

Soon after his death, people began reporting miracles at Anthony's tomb. The people of Padua, who had reviled him while he was alive, now tried to have him proclaimed a saint. The pope, however, said that one St. Anthony (of Padua) was enough for Padua. Nevertheless, he is known as Blessed Anthony Manzi, often called Blessed Anthony the Pilgrim.

Blessed Anthony Manzi's memorial is February 1.

8

St. Anthony Mary Pucci, O.S.M.
April 16, 1819 – January 12, 1892

EUSTACE PUCCI WAS BORN ON April 16, 1819, second of seven children, to a poor sacristan and his wife in Vernio, Italy.

From a very early age, Eustace had a desire to enter the priesthood, but his father was not very happy about this idea. However, when he was 18 years old, Eustace joined the Servite priory of the Annunciation in Florence. In the Religious life, he took the name Anthony Mary.

After studying at the Hermitage of Monte Senario near Florence, Anthony was ordained a priest in 1843 at the age of 24. He was appointed as curate of a new parish of St. Andrew in the seaside town of Viareggio, and four years later, he became pastor of the parish. It was in this parish that Fr. Anthony spent the rest of his life.

Although he was a good administrator, Fr. Anthony was most noted for his love for the people. He was especially noted for his compassion and sensitivity toward the poor, the sick, and the elderly.

Fr. Anthony's holiness especially shone to others during the epidemics of 1854 and 1866. In these epidemics, Fr. Anthony nursed the sick of the town. He also founded a seaside nursing home for children in the area, a very novel thing to do in those days.

Besides his pastoral work, including his nursing experiences, Fr. Anthony is noted for his part in founding the Holy Childhood Society. This society is now part of the Society for the Propagation of the Faith.

Fr. Anthony died on January 12, 1892 at the age of 72 in Viareggio, Italy. Pope St. John XXIII canonized him on December 9, 1962.
St. Anthony Mary Pucci's feast day is January 12.

9

Bl. Arnold Reche, F.S.C.
September 2, 1838 – October 23, 1890

NICHOLAS-JULES RECHE WAS BORN ON September 2, 1838 in northeastern France, eldest of eight children. His father was a poor shoemaker, and his mother was continually discontent because of the family's poverty.

Though Nicholas-Jules' parents had a troubled marriage, they did manage to ensure the children had a firm foundation in their Catholic Christian faith. Unfortunately, Nicholas-Jules' father was known as a "fanatic," and some of this strictness rubbed off on him. In his catechism class in his parish, the priest said that Nicholas-Jules was the only serious student in the class. Even as a youngster, Nicholas-Jules was noted for his piety and self-discipline.

When he was 21 years old, Nicholas-Jules became a coachman for a wealthy family, and then worked as a mule driver. More and more, he began to devote himself to prayer and to severe bodily austerities.

As a young man, he began helping the Brothers of the Christian Schools by teaching classes for teenagers. From this experience, Nicholas-Jules decided God was calling him to become a member of the Order. So in November 1862, he entered the novitiate of the Order, and on Christmas Day, he was clothed in the habit and took the name Brother Arnold. He made his simple vows in 1863 and final profession in 1871.

Although he spent fourteen years teaching at the Brothers' school in Reims, he was never very good at it. He had a difficult time keeping order in the classroom, perhaps because of his great kindness. This led him to see himself as a failure. He once wrote to a relative saying, "Pray for me that I may not be altogether useless, that I may accomplish all the good that God expects of me, that I won't be an obstacle to the good work that the Brothers around me are trying to do."

One area of his life where he did shine, however, was as a nurse in the Franco-Prussian War. In fact, his nursing service was so outstanding, that the International Red Cross awarded him a bronze cross for his nursing care of both French and German soldiers during the war.

Eventually, in 1877, his Order gave him the job of directing novices. This proved to be very rewarding for Brother Arnold, and he became known as an excellent spiritual director.

In March of 1890, Brother Arnold took over the job of director general of another house of the Brothers, even though he was in ill health. On October 23, 1890, he suffered a stroke and died after receiving the Sacrament of the Sick.

Pope St. John Paul II beatified him in November 1987.

Blessed Arnold's feast day is October 23rd.

10

St. Benedict of Nursia, O.S.B.
c. 480 – c. 550

BENEDICT WAS BORN IN NURSIA, Italy around 480. Though he has had enormous influence on many aspects of the Catholic Church, especially in the area of Western monasticism, not too much is known about specifics of his life. Rather, he is most famous because of his writings.

As a young man, Benedict went to Rome to study. However, he was so upset by what he considered to be the immorality of society that he gave up his schooling and went to live as a hermit in Subiaco.

Soon other men were attracted to him and became his disciples. Benedict arranged the men into 12 deaneries – small groups of 10 monks each – to live in a blend of monastic and eremitic (hermit) lifestyles. Monasticism is intrinsically social in nature, while the eremitic lifestyle is intrinsically solitary in nature.

Benedict stayed in Subiaco for 25 years. For reasons that are unclear, conflict arose in the community, and Benedict eventually left the area with a couple of monks and settled at Monte Cassino near Naples. It was at Monte Cassino that Benedict wrote – or finished writing – his famous Rule for monks.

Benedict was very close to his sister Scholastica, and the two of them had a close spiritual relationship. Benedict died about 550 and was buried next to his sister, St. Scholastica.

Although Benedict may never have actually practiced clinical nursing, he is included in this book because his Rule added to the body of nursing theory.

Benedict's Rule was very practical, moderate, and flexible. Monks and hermits have used his Rule to guide them through the ages. Some emphasize the social monastic vocation, while others focus more on the solitary hermit vocation.

We are interested in his Rule because of its Chapter 36 – "Of the Sick Brethren." In this chapter, Benedict begins by saying, "Above all things, care must be taken of the sick, that they be served in a very truth as Christ is served; because He hath said, 'I was sick and you visited me'" (Matthew 25: 36). For Benedict, serving the sick was serving Christ, for as Jesus said, "As long as you did it to one of these my least brethren, you did it to me" (Matthew 25: 40).

Benedict's model for the care of the sick was patient-centered. The sick were to receive special treatment. For example, while other monks were to abstain from certain foods such as meat, the sick were permitted to have these foods. The sick were to have more baths than other monks. Further, the monks who nursed the sick were to consider their nursing duties as a great honor of God.

Benedict, however, also knew human nature. He knew all about what today's sociologists call the "sick role." The sick role grants certain privileges to the patient, especially the right to be free from the responsibilities of adult social roles. Some patients fall in love with this role, and begin to "milk" their illness to take advantage of it. Therefore, Benedict reminded monks that when they are sick, they should not have "unnecessary demands." Further, once they are well, they need to return to their regular, monastic lifestyle.

Pope Honorius III canonized Benedict in 1220.

St. Benedict's feast day is July 11.

11

St. Benedict Menni, O.H.
March 11, 1841 – April 24, 1914

ANGELO ERCOLE MENNI-FIGINI WAS BORN on March 11, 1841 in Milan. His parents had a great sense of Catholic social teaching, especially the Christian commandments to help the sick and the poor.

After he graduated from high school in 1859, Angelo volunteered to help transport wounded soldiers who were returning from the battlefield to the hospital of the Brothers Hospitallers of St. John of God.

Angelo was so impressed by the nursing work of the Hospitallers, that he entered their Order. In Religious life, he took the name Benedict, and he was ordained a priest in 1866.

Fr. Benedict was clearly an extraordinary young man, for only a few months after his ordination, Pope Pius IX asked him to restore the Hospitaller Order in Spain that had been eliminated because of anti-clerical laws of the 1830s.

Fr. Benedict arrived in Barcelona in April of 1867. He knew very little Spanish, and he had no material goods. However, with the help of two Brothers, he began his work of restoring the Hospitaller Order in Spain.

In October of 1867, he opened a hospital for poor and abandoned children. This was especially helpful for children suffering from nutritional-deficiency related diseases such as scurvy and rickets.

In 1872, he became the Superior of the Order in Spain. However, in 1873, Spain once again introduced anti-clerical restrictions. To avoid death, he fled to Marseilles. There, he and some of the other members of his Order joined the Red Cross so that when the troubles in Spain ended, they could go back and continue their work. A Red Cross testimonial read, "During the war [Fr. Benedict Menni] carried everywhere both spiritual and physical assistance to the wounded without distraction of favor, and showing equal love and charity to both sides."

When the civil war in Spain ended, Fr. Benedict returned to Spain. He opened 17 psychiatric hospitals as well as other hospitals, not only in Spain but also in Mexico and Portugal. In 1884, his Order established a Spanish-American province, and he became the provincial.

In 1885, a cholera epidemic broke out in Madrid. Fr. Benedict and other members of the Order began to serve as nurses in many areas of the city. In addition to practicing bedside nursing care, Fr. Benedict had to teach his fellow Hospitallers basic nursing theory and practice. In addition, he taught the poor people of the city basic principles of hygiene. During this epidemic, then, Benedict found himself doing clinical nursing, public health nursing, and nursing education all at the same time.

In spite of all his administrative duties, Benedict always found time to nurse the sick. He especially was devoted to caring for children, people with polio, and the mentally ill. Fr. Benedict was especially present for the mentally ill – the "least of my brethren."

Because men nurses cared only for men in those days, Fr. Benedict was concerned that women did not get the same care. Therefore, he founded the Congregation of Hospitaller Sisters of the Sacred Heart of Jesus to care for women patients. The Church formally approved that Order in 1901.

From that time on, however, Fr. Benedict's life became increasingly filled with sorrow and problems. For example, a mentally ill woman in Madrid claimed he had abused her. This case, which went on for seven years, was finally thrown out of court.

Members of his Order were also angry with Benedict because many were jealous of the women Hospitallers, whom they saw as competition. Others in the Order were displeased when Benedict had to let some of the members of his Order go because of "doctrinal laxity."

Opposition against Fr. Benedict grew so strong, in fact, that the Hospitallers ordered him to leave Italy, and forbade him to live in any Hospitaller Sisters' houses in France.

After Benedict had a stroke and could no longer use his hand to write, the Order took away his secretary so he could no longer communicate with others.

Toward the end of his life, Benedict suffered from senile dementia. He died of a second stroke on April 24, 1914.

Pope St. John Paul II canonized him on November 21, 1999.

St. Benedict Menni's feast day is April 24.

St. Benedict Menni is a patron saint of the mentally ill as well as all sick persons.

12

Bl. Benito Solana Ruiz, C.P.
February 17, 1882 – July 25, 1936

BENITO SOLANA RUIZ WAS BORN on February 17, 1882 in Cintruénigo, Navarra. His father was the carpenter of the village.

Although his parents were not supportive of his desire to enter the Religious life, he entered the Passionist Order in Daimiel, Spain. Unfortunately, Benito was not a very good student, and had trouble with his seminary studies. Therefore, he became a Passionist Brother instead of a priest. In Religious life, he had the name "Benito of the Virgin of Villar."

In the Order, he held many jobs. In Daimiel, for example, he served as a cook and tailor. In 1919, he went to Cuba and served as a porter and tailor in the Passionist house in Santa Clara. In 1922, his superiors assigned him to the part of Mexico City called Tacubaya.

In those days, however, Mexico was in the throes of an anti-Catholic movement that came to be known as the *Cristero* War. For his safety, Brother Benito was sent back to Spain. Following a brief time in Daimiel, Benito began nursing the sick in Zaragoza.

As a Passionist Brother, Benito was known for his humility, charity and patience, especially when nursing sick patients.

On July 25, 1936, Benito was shot to death in Urdá, Toledo, a victim of the Spanish Civil War.

Pope St. John Paul II beatified Benito on October 1, 1989.

Blessed Benito Solana Ruiz' feast day is July 25.

13

Bl. Bentivoglio de Bonis, O.F.M.
1188 – December 25, 1232

BENTIVOGLIO WAS BORN IN SAN Severino Marche, Macerata, in the northeast of what is now Italy near the town of Assisi, in 1188. As an adult, he was called by God to follow the footsteps of St. Francis of Assisi, founder of the Franciscan Order. In fact, Bentivoglio became one of the first priests of the Order. Many of his relatives followed him and became Franciscans also.

According to reports from the parish priest of Severino and others, Bentivoglio was noted for his inspiring preaching ability, and his fervor and charity. The parish priest also claimed that he once saw Fr. Bentivoglio in ecstasy while praying in the woods.

The parish priest told how one day, Fr. Bentivoglio's superiors ordered him to move to a location fifteen miles from where he was living. Like a good Religious, Fr. Bentivoglio obeyed. However, Bentivoglio had been nursing a leper, and he did not want to abandon his nursing care. Therefore, legend has it that he carried the leper on his back to the new location so that he could continue nursing his patient. The story says, "…if [Bentivoglio] had been an eagle, he could not have flown in so short a time, and this divine miracle put the whole country round in amazement and admiration."

In addition to being noted as a nurse, priest and gifted preacher, some biographies call him a "miracle worker, healer, and visionary."

Fr. Bentivoglio died on Christmas Day, 1232, in his hometown of San Severino.

Pope Blessed Pius IX beatified Bentivoglio on December 30, 1852.

Blessed Bentivoglio's memorial day is December 25.

14

Bl. Benvenuto of Gubbio, O.F.M.
1100s – 1232

BENVENUTO WAS A KNIGHT OF Gubbio, Umbria, in what is now Italy. One day, he heard St. Francis of Assisi preaching. He was so captivated by Francis' preaching, that he presented himself to Francis and asked if he could become a follower of his.

Though Benvenuto could not read or write, he argued that as a knight, he would make a good Religious, as military men already had formed habits of discipline, endurance, and obedience.

Francis welcomed Benvenuto as a lay brother in the Order. Brother Benvenuto asked that he be allowed to work with the sick, and Francis granted his request. Soon, Brother Benvenuto found himself in charge of nursing lepers. Biographers of Benvenuto say he treated each leper as though he were treating Jesus himself. Brother Benvenuto practiced every form of nursing care for the lepers, and nothing was too repulsive for him to endure. He devoted his entire life to this care, waiting on his patients hand and foot. And even though he himself suffered from sicknesses, he bore his sufferings with saintly graciousness.

In addition to being an excellent nurse, Brother Benvenuto was known for his perfect obedience and prayer life. He would often be found spending the entire night in prayer, and he reportedly had frequent visions of the Child Jesus.

Brother Benvenuto died in Corneto – now known as Tarquinia –in 1232.

Pope Innocent XI beatified Benvenuto in 1697.

Blessed Benvenuto of Gubbio's feast day is June 25.

15

Bro. Bernardino de Obregón, O.M.
May 5, 1540 – August 6, 1599

BERNARDINO DE OBREGÓN WAS BORN on May 5, 1540 in Castile.

As a young adult, he became a soldier in the Spanish army. After his military service, Bernardino retired and dedicated his life to the care of the sick in various hospitals in Madrid. There he spent 20 years nursing the sick.

As time went on, other men joined Bernardino in his work. Bernardino not only taught these men nursing theory, he also gave them practical tips on clinical nursing practice. He also became the director of the general hospital in Madrid. Thus, Bernardino was not only a nurse clinician, he was also a nursing educator and administrator.

In 1567, the papal nuncio in Madrid approved Bernardino and his group of men nurses as a religious congregation. In addition to the traditional religious vows of poverty, chastity, and obedience, Bernardino's group took a fourth vow – free hospitality.

The new Order was known as the Minim Congregation of Poor Brothers Infirmarians, later simply known as the Obregonians. The Order did not found hospitals. Rather, they did their nursing service in already-established hospitals.

King Philip II entrusted the hospital of the Royal Court of Spain to the Brothers in the late 1500s. In 1592, Brother Bernardino and his congregation were invited by the Portuguese government to establish a facility there. So in 1592, the congregation founded an asylum for orphan boys.

In 1598, as King Philip II was nearing his death, Brother Bernardino was called back to Spain to be with the king. Bernadino, himself, died on August 6, 1599.

Although the Obregonian Order spread to other nations, it eventually disappeared. However, the Order is important in nursing history, for it was responsible for publication of the first manual for nursing care, written for nurses by a nurse. In 1617, Oregonian Brother Andrés Fernández published a book titled *Instrucción de Enfermeros y Método de Aplicar los Remedios a Todo Tipo de Enfermedades* – (*Training Nurses and a Method for Applying Remedies to All Forms of Illness*).

16
St. Bernardino of Siena, O.F.M.
September 8, 1380 – May 20, 1444

BERNARDINO WAS BORN TO A noble family on September 8, 1380 in Massa Marittima in what is now Italy.

Orphaned at the age of six, he was raised by a pious aunt.

In 1397, Bernardino received a degree in civil and canon law and joined the Confraternity of Our Lady that was attached to the hospital of Santa Maria della Scala church in Siena.

Three years later, a plague infected Siena. Bernardino immediately began to nurse the sick. When most of the regular nursing staff died, he took charge of the entire hospital with the help of ten of his companions. Bernardino nursed the sick for four months. Unfortunately, by the end of this time, Bernardino became sick from exhaustion.

As soon as he recovered, Bernardino began doing private duty nursing for his invalid aunt who had raised him. He nursed her until she died.

In 1402, Bernardino became a Franciscan, and two years later, he became a priest.

For more than 30 years, Fr. Bernardino made a name for himself as a very creative, entertaining, and powerful preacher all over Italy. He especially preached against gambling and vanity.

Unfortunately, Bernardino had two great faults: he was bigoted against Jews and gay men. Before we judge him too harshly for his bigotry, we must remember that in the day and culture in which he lived, such bigotry was not considered immoral.

Bernardino is also noted for his love of the Holy Name of Jesus. In fact, he designed a symbol – IHS – on a blazing sun. (The letters IHS are the first three letters of Jesus in Greek. This symbol is part of Pope Francis' coat-of-arms.)

Fr. Bernardino died on May 20, 1444 in Aquila, Italy when he was 63 years old.

Pope Nicholas V canonized him on May 24, 1450 in Rome.

St. Bernardino of Siena's feast day is May 20.

St. Bernardino of Siena is a patron saint of gambling addicts, advertisers, chest problems, public relations personnel, San Bernardino, California, and Aquila, Italy.

17

St. Bernard of Corleone, O.F.M. Cap.
February 6, 1605 – January 12, 1667

FILIPPO LATINO WAS BORN ON February 6, 1605 in Corleone, Sicily. His father, Leonardo, was a shoemaker in the town, and when Filippo was old enough, he learned the trade also. Another interesting fact about Filippo's childhood was that his home was known as the "house of saints." It got that reputation because Filippo's father frequently brought the needy to his home to wash, clothe, and feed them. Filippo, along with his brothers and sister, inherited this love for the poor in their hearts. At least in Filippo's case, this love and concern for those in need never left him.

Upon the death of his father, young Filippo became a soldier in the army. There he showed himself to have a fiery temper. And because he had become a very skilled swordsman, he often challenged men to fight him.

As a young soldier, Filippo had a reputation as a troublemaker and a man of loose morals. One day in 1624, when Filippo was 19, he wounded a challenger's hand. This caused the wounded man to lose his arm from infection. Though this was devastating to the victim, it was the turning point in Filippo's life. The incident shook him to the core of his being, and he began to change his life. He started by begging the victim's forgiveness, and eventually, the two became friends.

As time went on, Filippo became attracted to the Franciscan Capuchin friars. So when he was 31 years old, Filippo entered the novitiate of the

Capuchins in Caltanissetta on December 13, 1667. In Religious life, he took the name Bernard.

As a Capuchin friar, Bernard served as a lay brother. He abandoned his wild and fiery ways and replaced them with humility, obedience, and compassion. He also was unmercifully hard on his body, a type of spirituality that was considered acceptable in those days. For example, he would scourge himself several times a day to the point of drawing blood, and he slept only three hours per night on a board with a block of wood for a pillow. For most of his time as a friar, he limited his food intake to bread and water. If he had other food, he would put it in his mouth for the taste and then discard it. He also wore the shabbiest habits that were available in the friaries where he lived, and he would always ask for the most uncomfortable cell.

Brother Bernard served in many locations in his province, but the last fifteen years of his life he spent in Palermo.

As a friar, he had many jobs, but no matter what his assignment was, he had a deep love for caring for the sick, and he always found time for nursing those in need. He was noted to be a very gentle and compassionate nurse for friars in need.

Brother Bernard, in addition to nursing sick humans, also had a profound love for animals. In fact, he felt especially sorry for animals because they could not tell humans about what kind of pain they had and where it was located. Amazingly, however, God gave Brother Bernard the very special gift of healing animals. He was known as the "supernatural veterinary." People from far and wide would bring their sick animals to Brother Bernard. He would pray the Our Father, and then he would lead the animals around a cross in front of the Capuchin church three times. Then they would be cured. It is reported that on his deathbed, Brother Bernard "bequeathed" this gift of healing to another friar.

In addition to his regular duties, and to his nursing of humans and animals, Brother Bernard constantly helped other friars with their tasks to lighten their load. For example, Brother Bernard took over the care of all the other friars' laundry.

Brother Bernard died on January 12, 1667. On his deathbed, after receiving a blessing, he said, "Let's go, let's go." His good friend, Brother Antonino of Partanna, said that he saw Bernard's spirit repeating with joy, "Paradise! Paradise! O, blessed are the disciplines, blissful the night watches! Blessed the penances, the self-will sacrificed! O, the blessing of fasting, and acts of obedience! How great is the blessing of religious life well lived!"

Pope St. John Paul II canonized Bernardo on June 10, 2001.

St. Bernard of Corleone's feast day is January 12.

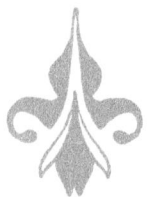

18

St. Bernardo Tolomei, O.S.B. Oliv.
May 10, 1272 – August 20, 1348

GIOVANNI TOLOMEI WAS BORN IN Siena, Tuscany on May 10, 1272.

His uncle Christopher, a Dominican priest, provided Giovanni with his early education. Though Giovanni wanted to enter the religious life from an early age, his father opposed his wishes.

Giovanni continued studying philosophy, mathematics, civil law, canon law, and theology. He was a knight in the armies of Rudolph I of Germany.

While studying law in Siena, Giovanni became a member of the Confraternity of the *Disciplinati di Santa Maria della Notte*, a group dedicated to serving the sick in the Hospital of Santa Maria della Scala. It is unclear whether Giovanni actually nursed the sick at this time, or if he served the sick in other ways. What is important, though, is that his membership in such a group showed a devotion to the sick as a young man. This love of the sick would come into play later in Giovanni's life during a time of plague.

In 1313, Giovanni and two companions from the Confraternity – Patrizio di Francesco Patrizi and Ambrogio di Nino Piccolomini – decided to live together as hermits on land in Accona that belonged to Giovanni's family. There they lived a life of manual labor, prayer, meditation, and silence. At that time, Giovanni changed his name to Bernardo in honor St. Bernard of Clairvaux, a Cistercian abbot.

At the end of 1318 or the beginning of 1319, Bernardo had a vision of monks clad in white robes climbing a ladder, helped by angels, to Jesus and

Mary. Bernardo interpreted this as a divine sign that he was supposed to found a religious community.

After receiving permission from the bishop of Arezzo in March of 1319 to build a monastery, Bernardo and his men began building the monastery of Santa Maria di Monte Oliveto. Bernardo made monastic vows, and took a white robe like the white habits of Camaldolese hermits and Carthusian and Cistercian monks. They also adopted the Rule of St. Benedict with certain modifications.

Bernardo, much against his nature, became the fourth abbot of the monastery and remained so until his death. His branch of the Benedictines is frequently called the Order of Our Lady of Mount Olivet or, more commonly, the Olivetans.

In 1346, a plague came to Siena. Bernardo and his monks left the solitude of Monte Oliveto and went to the monastery of San Benedetto a Porta Tufi in Siena where they could live temporarily while nursing the sick of the city. During the plague, Bernardo and his fellow monks served valiantly as nurses caring for plague victims. Unfortunately, Bernardo and many other monks caught the plague. Bernardo died on August 20, 1384 from nursing the plague victims. Eighty-four other monks also died.

In 1735, an Italian painter named Giuseppe Maria Crespi painted a work called "Blessed Bernard Tolomei Interceding for the Cessation of the Plague in Siena."

Pope Benedict XVI canonized Bernardo Tolomei on April 26, 2009.

St. Bernardo Tolomei's feast day is August 20.

19

St. Cajetan, C.R.
October 1, 1480 – August 7, 1547

CAJETAN WAS BORN TO A noble family on October 1, 1480 in Vicenza, Lombardy.

When he was 24 years old, Cajetan received a doctorate in civil and canon law. He became a senator of Vicenza, and in 1506 went to work as a diplomat for Pope Julius II.

When the Pope died in 1513, Cajetan left the papal court and prepared for the priesthood. In 1516, Cajetan was ordained a priest.

While Fr. Cajetan was in Rome, he helped co-found the Oratory of the Divine Love. This was a confraternity of priests who tried to live holy lives. In time, Fr. Cajetan would found or become associated with other Oratories. Unfortunately, many of his friends looked down on Cajetan because some of the oratories with which he was associated attracted men from very poor backgrounds, quite unlike his own noble background. His friends, therefore, felt that Cajetan was disgracing his family's honor.

Around 1520, Cajetan began a major work of nursing the sick. In 1522, he founded a hospital for incurables in his hometown of Vicenza, and in 1523, he founded a hospital in Venice. The importance of his nursing experience was seen when Cajetan said that in his Oratory, the men tried to serve God by worship, but "in our hospital we can say that we actually find him."

Though he focused on nursing the sick, Fr. Cajetan was very distracted by the laxity of the clergy of his day. So on September 14, 1524, Cajetan joined with three other men to found a new Order of priests called the Canons Regular. Eventually, the Order would be known as the Theatines. The new Order wanted to help priests live a holier lifestyle, a lifestyle based on studies, preaching, pastoral care, and better liturgy. The members of the Order also wanted to devote themselves to nursing the sick.

In 1527, the army of Charles V sacked Rome, and the Theatines' house was destroyed. The Theatines fled to Venice, where in 1530, they nursed the victims of a plague and subsequent famine.

After many years of nursing and fighting for a holier priesthood, Fr. Cajetan died in Naples on August 7, 1547.

Pope Clement V canonized him on April 12, 1671.

St. Cajetan's feast day is August 7.

St. Cajetan is a patron saint of workers, gamblers, job seekers, and the nations of Albania, Italy, Malta, Argentina, Brazil, El Salvador, and Guatemala.

20

St. Camillus de Lellis, M.I.
May 25, 1550 – July 14, 1614

CAMILLUS WAS BORN IN NAPLES on May 25, 1550 in Bucchianico, Naples.

When he was 16 or 17 years old, he followed in his father's footsteps by becoming a soldier. Camillus was a huge man, six feet six inches tall, and he had a very fiery temper. As a soldier, he lived a wild lifestyle of drinking and brawling and getting into all kinds of trouble. His biggest problem, however, was his addiction to gambling.

When he was 21, Camillus was admitted to a hospital in Rome because of a leg ulcer that never did heal. Because he was so quarrelsome, he was expelled from the hospital. So he went back to being a soldier.

By the time he was 24, Camillus' gambling addiction caused him to lose everything, even the shirt off his back. Reduced to a pauper, Camillus remembered a vow he had made earlier in life to become a Franciscan. The Franciscans took him in as a laborer, but they let him go because of his incurable leg ulcer.

When he was 25, Camillus returned to the hospital where he had worked a few years earlier, and there he began an amazing transformation. He began to care for the sick as a nurse. When he saw what poor nursing care was being given, he became incredibly angry, and set out to make some changes. He proved to be a spectacular nurse, and eventually became the hospital administrator.

During Camillus' time in the hospital, he also studied for the priesthood and was ordained when he was 34 years old.

Camillus founded his own hospital, and he attracted men who also had a devotion to serving God by serving others who were sick. This group of men eventually became known as the Ministers of the Sick, priests and brothers who served the sick physically and spiritually. These men wore a large red Latin cross on their habits and on their capes.

Camillus and his followers had a special love for prisoners, people suffering from the plague, and soldiers. Some of the Ministers of the Sick, who eventually came be known as the Camillian Fathers and Brothers, cared for plague victims. Many became contaminated by the plague and died. Others were sent to battlefields in Hungary and Croatia to care for the sick.

Camillus instituted many modern nursing practices such as proper ventilation, good nutrition, and isolating persons with contagious diseases. Many of his principles are taught even today in schools of nursing.

Camillus insisted that his priests and brothers see Christ in every sick person. He insisted on what he called "old-fashioned charity but with up-to-date technical skill." His guiding principle was the maxim of Jesus, "Whatever you did for one of these least brothers of mine, you did for me" (Mt 25: 40). At the time of his death on July 14, 1614, he had established fifteen houses of his congregation and eight hospitals.

Pope Benedict XIV canonized Camillus in 1746.

St. Camillus' feast day in the United States is July 18.

St. Camillus is a patron saint of nurses, nursing administrators, hospitals, physicians, the sick, and those suffering from gambling addiction.

21

St. Carthach (Mo Chutu) of Lismore
Died May 14, 639

CARTHACH, ALSO KNOWN AS Mo Chutu, was an Irish monk, hermit, and nurse. The exact date of his birth is unknown.

He came from a wealthy family and helped tend livestock as a child. One day, the story goes, he heard some monks chanting as they passed by in procession. He was so touched that he decided to become a monk himself.

After Carthach was a monk for some time, a bishop ordained him a priest. Around 590, Fr. Carthach founded a group of monks in County Kerry but was driven out by anti-clerical forces.

After visiting other monasteries, Fr. Carthach founded another monastery in 595. He also wrote a Rule for his monks. In addition to guiding monks on how to live, he also made recommendations on how bishops, priests, and kings should live their lives.

Eventually, Carthach became a bishop. As a bishop, he founded a hospital for lepers where he and his fellow monks did the nursing. After 40 years of caring for the sick, he and his fellow monks were expelled from their monastery by jealous religious and civil authorities. They did not abandon their patients, however, but rather took them along. Bishop Carthach founded a new installation for his monks and patients around 636 in Lismore, County Waterford. St. Carthach is considered to be the founder of the Diocese of Lismore.

Because of the hectic nature of building a new facility, Carthach decided he needed more peace and quiet. Therefore, he left the community to become a hermit on the Blackwater River.

When it was time for Carthach to die, the monks of Lismore carried him back to the monastery he had founded. He died peacefully on May 14, 639 near a cross that has come to be known as "the migration cross."

The last hospital and monastery that he founded flourished into the Middle Ages.

St. Carthach's feast day is May 15th.

22

St. Charles of Sezze, O.F.M.
October 19, 1613 – January 6, 1670

GIANCARLO MARCHIONI WAS BORN ON October 19, 1613 in Sezze, Papal States, to a poor farm family.

When he was a child, his mother liked to dress him as a friar in honor of St. Francis of Assisi and St. Anthony of Padua. His maternal grandmother provided Giancarlo with a strong foundation in the Catholic faith.

As a youth, Giancarlo helped his family by working as a shepherd on the farm and plowing the fields. He developed a desire to become a missionary in India, but his health was never adequate for the missionary life. He was also greatly inspired by the lives of two Franciscan Brothers – St. Paschal Baylon and St. Salvador of Horta (who is one of the Saintly Men of Nursing in this book).

In 1630, when he was about 17 years old, Giancarlo made a private vow of chastity. In 1633, he became so ill that death was a definite possibility. He vowed that if God spared his life, he would become a Franciscan friar.

Giancarlo's life was indeed spared. Though his parents very much wanted him to study for the priesthood, he could barely read or write because he did not receive a solid academic foundation as a child.

Giancarlo joined the Order of Friars Minor at Nazzano in 1635 and made his solemn profession as a Franciscan Brother on May 19, 1636. Though he wanted to take the name of "Cosmos" in Religious life, he bowed to his mother's insistence that it be "Carlo" (Charles) instead.

Brother Carlo served in many friaries as a cook, sacristan, gardener, porter, and beggar. Though he tried to do his best, he did not always excel at what he did. One person, for example, called Brother Carlo "an accident waiting to happen." This judgment might have come from the fact that he once started a huge fire in the kitchen when the oil he was using to fry onions burst into flames.

Although Brother Carlo was not a priest, his holiness was well known not only in the friaries in which he served, but also outside the Franciscan community. Indeed, popes Innocent X and Clement IX sought out Brother Carlo for counseling.

Although he was not officially assigned as an infirmarian in the friaries, Brother Carlo made a name for himself by nursing the sick in Carpineto when an epidemic of cholera ravaged the area.

The final and most fascinating event in Brother Carlo's life occurred in late 1669 and early 1670. As Pope Clement IX lay dying in the first week of December 1669, he asked that Brother Carlo come to him. Because Brother Carlo was so ill himself, Carlo's fellow friars had to carry him on a chair to the pope. The pope insisted that Brother Carlo bless him, and the good friar did just that.

When Carlo was about to leave, the pope asked when the two would meet again. Brother Carlo assured him that they would meet again on the Feast of the Epiphany, January 6.

The pope, however, died on December 9, 1669. Everyone thought that Brother Carlo had been incorrect in predicting that he and the pope would meet on the Epiphany. But when Brother Carlo died on the Feast of the Epiphany, 1670, everyone realized that indeed, the two men were meeting in heaven on that very day.

Pope St. John XXIII canonized Carlo on April 12, 1959.

St. Charles of Sezze's feast day is January 6.

He is a patron saint of Sezze and of the Diocese of Latina-Teracina-Sezze-Priverno in Italy.

23

St. Crispin of Viterbo, O.F.M. Cap
November 13, 1668 – May 19, 1750

PIETRO FIORETTI WAS BORN IN Viterbo, Papal States on November 13, 1668 to a poor family. His mother dedicated him to the Blessed Virgin Mary when he was only a young child.

From a young age, people in the community began calling him "the little saint" because he was so pious and had such knowledge of the saints. His uncle taught him to be a shoemaker.

After being educated by Jesuits, Pietro entered the Capuchin Franciscan order as a lay brother in Viterbo. He took the name Crispin in Religious life because St. Crispin was a patron saint of shoemakers.

In the community, Brother Crispin served as a gardener and cook. Eventually, he was sent to the town of Tolfa and was given the job of infirmarian, or nurse, of the Capuchin community.

When an epidemic came to the area, Brother Crispin nursed the sick heroically. Many of his patients believed that their cure was the result of his prayers.

Though he was a simple lay brother, his fame spread. Cardinals, bishops, and even a pope came to visit him.

After serving in many of the Capuchin houses, he was sent to Orvieto. In that community, he served as the *questor*, the person whose job it was to beg for alms to support the religious community. Brother Crispin was so successful at his begging, that the housewives of the community fell in love with him and were always glad to see him. One day, his superiors decided that he needed an easier job in the community. This made the housewives of the town so upset that they refused to even speak to Crispin's replacement. The superiors knew they had to give Crispin his job as *questor* back; it was either that, or they would starve.

Brother Crispin liked to call himself the "ass or beast of burden of the Capuchins." Once, when a stranger asked him why he was not wearing a hat or hood, Crispin replied, "An ass does not wear a hat."

Brother Crispin spent his last years in Rome. In Rome, he was known for his wise sayings, prophecies, and multiplication of food (in the sense of the Miracle of the Loaves and Fishes). He also taught the basics of the Catholic faith to mountain peasants.

Brother Crispin died on May 19, 1750 in Rome at the age of 81.

Pope St. John Paul II canonized Crispin on June 20, 1982. His was John Paul II's first canonization.

St. Crispin of Viterbo's feast day is December 15.

24

St. Damien of Molokai, SS.CC.
January 3, 1840 – April 15, 1889

Jozef De Veuster was born the seventh child of a Flemish corn merchant and his wife on January 3, 1840 in Tremelo in Belgium. The faith of his family was quite strong: two of his sisters became Religious Sisters, and Jozef and his brother Auguste became priests.

Jozef had to quit school when he was 13 to work on the family farm. When he was 19, he entered the Congregation of the Sacred Hearts of Jesus and Mary. In Religious life, he took the name Damien. His brother Auguste, known as Fr. Pamphile in Religious life, was also a member of this Order, which is often known as the Picpus congregation.

When Damien first entered the Order on October 7, 1860, his superiors felt he was destined to be a Brother because of his lack of formal education. However, his brother tutored him, and eventually Damien was able to study for the priesthood. During his seminary studies, he prayed every day before a picture of the great missionary, St. Francis Xavier (who is a Saintly Man of Nursing in this book), that one day he would be given the honor of being a missionary.

Three years after entering the Picpus Order, Damien got his wish. Because his brother Pamphile was unable to take a missionary assignment to Hawaii, Damien was permitted to take his place.

On March 19, 1864, Damien landed in Honolulu Harbor and on May 21, 1864, Damien was ordained a priest.

Fr. Damien's first assignment was on the island of Hawaii, but in 1873, he volunteered to serve in the Hawaiian government's leper colony in Kalaupapa on the island of Molokai.

Initially, the plan was for four priests to serve on Molokai for three months each year. But when Fr. Damien went there, he fell in love with the people and the place. He was indeed like the proverbial "kid in a candy store" with unlimited opportunities to do mission work. Molokai was a missionary's dream.

In those days, lepers were treated horribly. Once a person was diagnosed with leprosy, he or she was taken by boat and thrown overboard once the boat got near Molokai. At that point, the leper had to swim to shore or drown.

When Fr. Damien first encountered the more than 800 lepers in the colony, he was appalled. The sight of rotten toes and fingers and noses was horrifying, and the stench of the wounds was worse. However, Damien began to get used to the sights and smells, and soon he found himself nursing the sick as best he could. He also made coffins and dug graves when members of his flock died.

Fr. Damien knew, however, that he also had to get busy building for the people. Soon, with the people's help, he built new houses, an orphanage, a clinic, a school, a church, and eventually a hospital. He even built furniture for the people's houses. He dedicated his parish to St. Philomena. He also helped people set up farms on the island, and he built a reservoir for a steady water supply.

In addition to his nursing and building, Fr. Damien was a one-man crusader for better conditions for the inhabitants of Molokai, demanding the Hawaiian government do more. His efforts paid off when the government did finally begin to become more active.

Fr. Damien, like Saint Teresa of Calcutta, was well known worldwide for his work and holiness long before his death. Fortunately, this notoriety helped recruit help for Fr. Damien's work.

In 1883, Sister Marianne Cope (now Saint Marianne of Molokai), along with six other Sisters of St. Francis of Syracuse, New York came to Molokai to help Fr. Damien. Soon, the Sisters had a hospital running.

In 1886, Joseph Dutton – more commonly known as "Brother Joseph" (and one of the Saintly Men of Nursing in this book) – arrived to help Fr. Dutton. Joseph was such a blessing that on his deathbed, Fr. Damien told everyone that he could die in peace, knowing Brother Joseph was there to take his place.

Eventually Fr. Damien contacted leprosy himself. One of the persons who came to help him was James Sinnett, a nurse from Mercy Hospital in Chicago. Sinnett, called "Brother James" by Fr. Damien, served as Fr. Damien's secretary in Damien's final days and nursed him to the very end.

Fr. Damien died on April 15, 1889 at the age of 49.

When Hawaii became a state of the United States of America in 1959, it chose Damien as one of its two representatives in the Statuary Hall in the U.S. Capitol.

Pope Benedict XVI canonized Damien on October 11, 2009.

St. Damien of Molokai's feast day is May 10.

St. Damien is a patron saint of persons with Hansen's Disease (leprosy).

25

St. Didacus (Diego), O.F.M.
1400 – November 12, 1463

DIDACUS, ALSO KNOWN AS DIEGO, was born to a poor family some time in 1400 in the town of San Nicolás del Puerto in the Archdiocese of Seville.

As a young person, he felt called to the vocation of a hermit. When he became friends with an older priest-hermit, Didacus placed his spiritual life under him. Together, the two hermits busied themselves with prayer, cultivating a garden and making wooden dishes, baskets, and other useful utensils. And like his spiritual director, he engaged in austerities often found in the spiritual lives of many Religious in those days and times.

After some years of living the hermit lifestyle, Didacus joined the Franciscan house at Arrizafa and became a lay brother. After profession of vows, Didacus was sent to the Canary Islands where his Order worked to meet the spiritual needs of the people. For example, in addition to being the porter or doorkeeper of the house, he found time to help with catechizing people in the Catholic faith.

In 1445, his superiors appointed Brother Didacus to be the Guardian of the Franciscan community on the Island of Fuerteventura, site of the Monastery of St. Bonaventure. Giving a simple lay brother this honor was highly unusual, so it shows that Didacus was not just an ordinary friar. Rather, his superiors must have detected leadership potential in this man.

In 1450, Brother Didacus joined fellow friars in traveling to Rome, where Pope Nicholas V had declared a Jubilee Year. The friars were eager to attend the canonization of Bernardino of Siena (one of the Saintly Men of Nursing in this book).

Unfortunately, the travelers from different nations brought with them various infections, and soon an epidemic broke out in Rome.

Always ready to help where needed, Brother Didacus threw himself into nursing the sick at the friary attached to the Basilica of Santa Maria in Ara Coeli, Rome. Not only did he distinguish himself as a nurse, but also miraculous cures as a result of his prayers soon began to be reported.

After the epidemic was over, his superiors called Brother Didacus back to Spain. There, he lived the last 13 years of his life enjoying a serene life among fellow friars. Brother Didacus died peacefully on November 12, 1463 in the friary at Alcalá, Spain.

Pope Sixtus V canonized him in 1588.

St. Didacus' feast day in the United States is November 12.

26

Bl. Edward J.M. Poppe
December 18, 1890 – June 10, 1924

EDWARD JOANNES MARIA POPPE WAS born on December 18, 1890 in Temse, Belgium. He was one of 11 children, son of a baker and his wife. The family was very devout: one of his brothers was a priest, and five of his sisters were Religious Sisters.

In spite of having so many siblings, Edward received an excellent education including studying at the Catholic University of Louvain.

As a seminarian, he was drafted into the army in World War I. Many of his fellow soldiers ridiculed him because he was a seminarian. Nevertheless, he weathered their hazing and became a good soldier. In fact, he served as a nurse on the battlefield in the war. Many of his fellow soldiers became convinced that because of his prayers to St. Joseph, many prisoners of war were freed miraculously. Needless to say, that made him a hero to many.

After he left the military, Edward became a priest on May 1, 1916. He took, as his motto, *"Accendatur,"* which means, "May the fire be kindled."

After ordination, Edward served as an associate pastor of Sint-Coleta, a poor parish in Ghent. Because so many of his parishioners were poor laborers, Fr. Edward chose to live his life in severe poverty to demonstrate his identification with them. In this parish, he devoted his time to the poor, the sick, and the dying. He also loved children and taught them catechism.

Unfortunately, Fr. Edward's health was never good, and together with his severe lifestyle, he became very weak. As a result, he was transferred to rural Moerzeke, where he lived from 1918 to 1922.

In May of 1919, he had a heart attack and was sent to a monastery to recover. While in the monastery, he threw himself into writing thousands of letters and articles, many of them against materialism and Marxism. Many of his articles appeared in a popular youth magazine of the day—*Zonneland*.

During this time, Fr. Edward also developed a special devotion to St. Therese of Lisieux, the "Little Flower." He tried to follow her "little way" of spirituality.

After his health seemed to improve, Fr. Edward became a spiritual director at a military school in Leopoldsburg in 1922. While he was visiting his mother at Christmastime, 1923, he had a cardiac crisis. As a result of this, he had to return to the monastery in Moerzeke. Edward had a heart attack in January of 1924, and six months later, he died of a stroke on June 10, 1924 at the monastery.

On October 2, 1999, Pope St. John Paul II beatified him.

Blessed Edward Poppe's feast day is June 10.

27

Bl. Engelmar Unzeitig, C.M.M.
March 1, 1911 – March 2, 1945

HUBERT UNZEITIG (THE NAME MEANS "unseasonable") was born on March 1, 1911 in Greifendorf, Bohemia (now part of the Czech Republic).

When he was 18 years old, he joined the Congregation of the Missionaries of Marianhill. In 1939, he was ordained a priest of that Order and took the name Engelmar in consecrated life.

While in parish ministry, the Gestapo arrested him on April 21, 1941 for being a Catholic priest and for preaching against Hitler's Nazi regime. He was 30 years old. After his arrest, Fr. Engelmar was sent to the Dachau concentration camp, where he would spend the next four years of his life.

Dachau was once described as the "largest Catholic cemetery for priests in the world" because over 2,500 Catholic seminarians, priests, and Religious were sent there, and over 1,000 died there.

In the camp, Fr. Engelmar did all he could to help the other inmates. He studied Russian, for example, so he could better serve prisoners coming from Eastern Europe.

Once he wrote a letter that said, in part, "Even behind the hardest sacrifices and worst suffering stands God with his fatherly love, who is satisfied with the good will of his children and gives them and others happiness."

When a typhoid epidemic broke out in Dachau, Fr. Engelmar, along with 19 other Catholic priests, volunteered to do nursing in the typhoid barrack. Fr. Engelmar's volunteering was no surprise, for it was not only in harmony with his ever-ready desire to serve, it was also in harmony with his Congregation's motto: "If no one else will go, I will go."

Of the 20 priests who served as nurses for the typhoid patients, all but two died from typhoid. Fr. Engelmar was one of them, dying on March 2, 1945. Fr. Engelmar is often known as "The Angel of Dachau."

Pope Benedict XVI proclaimed him "Venerable" on July 3, 2009. On January 21, 2016, Pope Francis proclaimed that Venerable Engelmar's death was martyrdom, making the path to beatification much easier.

On September 24, 2016, Pope Francis beatified Engelmar.

Blessed Engelmar Unzeitig's feast day is March 2.

28

Bl. Enrico Rebuchini, M.I.
April 25, 1860 – May 9 or 10, 1938

ENRICO REBUCHINI WAS BORN ON April 25, 1860 near Lake Como in the town of Gravedona, Italy. His family was wealthy. Though his mother was a devout Catholic Christian, his father was not at all in favor of religion. Though Enrico's father would accompany his wife to church, he would remain outside during the services.

From an early age, Enrico felt a strong call to the priesthood, the Religious life, or both. Unfortunately, because of his father's opposition, he sought to find an occupation as a layperson. First, he enrolled at the University of Pavia to study mathematics, but he left after a year because did not like the anticlericalism he found there.

When he returned to Como, he studied at the Military School at Milan, and he graduated as a reserve second lieutenant. His superiors, greatly impressed with him, wanted him to make a career in the army. He declined their wishes, however, and returned home to study accounting. In 1882 he received his diploma.

After graduation, Enrico entered his brother-in-law's silk business. Though he was competent in his work, he became very depressed at not being to pursue a vocation in religion. Depression would afflict him on and off for the rest of his life.

In the summer of 1884, however, Saint Luigi Guanella asked the monks of all the monasteries of Como to pray for Enrico's vocation. At last, his father agreed to give Enrico his blessing, and Enrico entered the Gregorian University in Rome to study to become a priest.

Unfortunately, Enrico was not prudent in his spiritual life, and this led him to excessive penances. Soon, he entered a period of "profound nervous depression" that lasted from March 1886 to May 1887. He had to leave his studies and return home to recover.

In May of 1887, Enrico recovered, and in the summer of 1887, he found a job at a hospital in Como. It was there that Enrico developed a profound love for the sick. In fact, he spent every spare minute nursing the sick, especially the poor, the neediest, and the most isolated. He spent every cent he had on them, and he even visited the sick in their homes. Unfortunately, however, this was not the job for which he was hired, so he was soon graciously fired.

At last, Enrico had found his passion. Having heard about the Servants of the Sick that had been founded by the great nurse-priest St. Camillus de Lellis (another Saintly Man of Nursing in this book), he joined the Camillians on September 27, 1887 at the age of 27.

Soon Enrico developed a reputation for his good-naturedness. Because of his personality, and because of his previous extensive studies, Bishop Sarto of Mantua – later to be known as Pope St. Pius X – ordained him on April 14, 1889 during his novitiate. Fr. Enrico took his final profession on December 8, 1891.

From his ordination until 1899, Fr. Enrico worked at Verona's civil and military hospital and then, from 1903 to 1937, he was the administrator of the St. Camillus clinic in Cremona. Though much of Enrico's life as a Camillian Father was spent working with plumbing, electrical failures, roof repairs, and other mundane activities, his true passion was nursing the sick.

During his lifetime, people in the streets came to know Fr. Enrico as a very special person. In fact, the people called him the "mystic of the streets."

Even to the end of his life, Fr. Enrico served the sick. For example, just a few days before his death, he celebrated Mass for a sick person. Afterwards, he became sick and died on May 9 or 10, 1938 from pneumonia.

Pope St. John Paul II beatified Enrico on May 4, 1997.

Blessed Enrico Rebuschini's feast day is May 10.

29

St. Fidelis of Sigmaringen, O.F.M. Cap.
1577 – April 24, 1622

MARK ROY, OR REY, WAS born sometime in 1577 in Sigmaringen in what is now Germany.

As a young man, he studied law at the University of Freiburg. As a college student, Mark exhibited certain qualities that foreshadowed his later attraction to the Religious life. For example, he abstained from wine, wore a hair shirt, and was noted for the virtues of chastity and humility.

After graduation, he taught philosophy at the same university. In 1604, he took a small group of aristocratic students on a trip all over Western Europe. While traveling, Mark not only served the young men as a guide, he also taught them to treasure their Catholic Faith and to care for the poor that they met on their journey.

In 1611, Mark obtained a Doctor of Law degree in civil and canon law. After obtaining his degree, he began practicing law. Soon, he became known as "the poor man's lawyer" because of his love of the poor and his readiness to help them in spite of their lack of money.

After practicing law for a while, however, Mark became disillusioned by the questionable practices of his fellow lawyers. Therefore, he decided to leave law and become a priest.

Mark joined his brother, George, who was in the Franciscan Capuchin Order. In Religious life, Mark took the name Fidelis, which in English means

"Faithful." He gave away his money to needy seminarians and the poor, and was eventually ordained a priest.

As a priest, he spent much of his time preaching and celebrating Reconciliation. Soon, he became known for his holiness, prayer life, and austerities.

From 1614 to 1618, he studied theology.

As a priest, Fr. Fidelis was not only a capable administrator of the friaries in which he lived, but was also a powerful preacher who converted many Protestants to the Catholic Faith.

But no matter in what type of ministry Fidelis found himself, he always had a special devotion to the poor and the sick. During a very severe epidemic, for example, he distinguished himself as an excellent nurse, nursing sick soldiers. Many of the soldiers that Fr. Fidelis cared for believed that it was through his nursing care that God performed miraculous cures.

Fr. Fidelis died on April 24, 1622.

Pope Benedict XIV canonized him on June 29, 1746.

St. Fidelis of Sigmaringen's feast day is April 24.

30

St. Finnian of Clonard
470 – December 12, 549

FINNIAN WAS BORN AROUND 470 in Myshall, a town of County Carlow in Ireland. His father was a nobleman.

As with many saints of old times, there were legends associated with Finnian. For example, many said that when Finnian was an infant, his mother had a dream that all the birds of Ireland gathered together to show that her son would be a very holy person.

St. Abban, an Irish hermit, baptized Finnian. And when Finnian was quite young, his parents placed him under the direction of Bishop Forchern of Trim in the Diocese of Meath. Some historians believe Finnian studied in Gaul (now France) and Wales.

Where he studied is not so important. What is important is that Finnian became a monk and established many monasteries and churches in Ireland. His most famous monastery was on the banks of the Boyne River at Clonard in County Meath. It was in this monastery that three thousand men came to learn from him. Because of his great influence on the Irish monastic world of his time, Finnian became known as the "Teacher of the Saints of Ireland." He was especially noted for his love and insight into Bible studies.

Around 549, the plague hit Clonard, and Finnian busied himself nursing the sick. This he did until he himself contracted the plague from his patients. As a result of his nursing, Finnian died in on December 12, 549.

St. Finnian's feast day is December 12.

St. Finnian is a patron saint of the Diocese of Meath in Ireland.

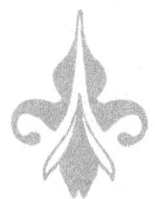

31

St. Francis of Assisi, O.F.M.
1181 – October 3, 1226

OF ALL THE SAINTS IN the Catholic Church, St. Francis of Assisi is one of the most popular and well recognized. He is usually pictured wearing the brown habit of Franciscan friars with a bird on his finger and animals at his feet.

Giovanni di Pietro Bernardone was born sometime in 1181 in Assisi. His father was a successful merchant. Both his mother and father were Catholic Christians who passed on the faith to Giovanni.

When his father returned to Assisi from a business trip to France, he added the name "Francesco" to his son's name. In English-speaking countries, the son has come to be known as Francis.

Like many young men of his time who had plenty of money, Francis loved to party and host lavish banquets for his friends. He also dreamed of one day becoming a knight and living a chivalrous life. Therefore, when he was 20 years old, he enlisted in the war between Assisi and Perugia.

In the war, Francis was captured and spent a year in captivity. When he was finally released, he was struck down by a serious illness – possibly malaria - that lasted about a year. Still considering himself a soldier, he volunteered to fight once again. In fact, he wanted to follow a Count named Walter of Brienne whom, he hoped, would make him a knight. That was not to happen, for when he got to a place called Spoleto, he learned Count Walter had died. This led Francis into depression and a recurrence of his malaria.

It was in Spoleto that Francis had a strange dream that told him to follow the Master, not the servant. He interpreted this to mean he was to follow

God, not Walter. This was the beginning of a dramatic conversion experience for Francis.

One day, as Francis was traveling on his horse, he saw a leper. Now Francis had a great revulsion toward lepers, but on this occasion, he dismounted from his horse, went up to the leper, and kissed the leper's hand. Francis began nursing lepers from that time on, in houses and hospitals, when he had free time. He attributed his nursing experience as the most significant event of his conversion.

Some time later, Francis heard another voice saying, "Francis, rebuild my church." Francis at first thought the message was to repair a neighborhood church building called San Damiano. Only later did he come to believe the message was to be a reformer of the Catholic Church at large.

Although it made Francis' father very angry, Francis renounced his inheritance and turned his back on things of the world. After stripping himself naked and giving his father the clothes on his back, he put on a laborer's smock and dedicated himself to poverty.

For the next two years, Francis lived as a recluse and spent time nursing the sick, especially those who were poor, and begging for alms to support his work.

Soon, other men were attracted to Francis and wanted to share in the new mendicant life he was living. This led to the creation of the Order of Friars Minor. Later, St. Clare of Assisi and other women would also come to follow him and form their own branch of Franciscans.

Brother Francis never felt worthy to be ordained a priest, but he did consent to be ordained a deacon.

Francis died on October 3, 1226.

Pope Gregory IX canonized Francis of Assisi on July 16, 1228.

St. Francis of Assisi's feast day is October 4.

St. Francis of Assisi is a patron saint of animals; the environment and environmentalists; San Francisco, California; Naga City, Cebu, Philippines; tapestry workers; and the many branches of the extended Franciscan family.

32

St. Francis Mary of Camporosso, O.F.M. Cap.
December 27, 1804 – September 17, 1866

GIOVANNI CROESE WAS BORN ON December 27, 1804, fourth of five children, in Camporosso on the Ligurian coast of what is now Italy. His father was a farm worker in an olive orchard. All of the children of the family were expected to do their share of chores, and they received simple but pious educations.

When he was 18 years old, Giovanni met a Conventual Franciscan lay brother who inspired him to join the Order. Giovanni was accepted into the community in Sestri Ponente, outside of Genoa, and given the name Antonio.

After two years, Brother Antonio decided he desired to live in a community with a more austere life. Therefore, he left the Conventual Franciscans and joined a Capuchin Franciscan community. In 1825, he made his profession as a lay brother and was given the name Francisco Maria (Francis Mary).

In his new life, Brother Francis Mary worked in the infirmary of the friary as a nurse. He was also given the job of *questor*, a person who begs in the streets for alms to support the friars.

At first, the people of Genoa made fun of him. Anti-religious bigots abused him, as did common neighborhood bullies. Nevertheless, Brother Francis Mary persevered for 40 years.

In time, he became highly popular, especially in the dockyards. People discovered that Brother Francis Mary had an amazing gift of knowing things about people that nobody else knew. For example, he could tell dock workers about the welfare of their loved ones who lived far away.

In time, the residents of Genoa began calling him "Padre Santo" or "Holy Father" even though he was not a priest.

In 1866, a cholera epidemic devastated Genoa. Brother Francis Mary did not hesitate to begin nursing the sick, even though he suffered from varicose veins. Though he was an excellent nurse, the hospital staff believed he was too frail to be doing that work.

As a result, Brother Francis Mary left the hospital and began doing what would now be called psychosocial nursing in the streets for the poor. On occasion, he also did ordinary physical nursing on the streets when needed.

Brother Francis Mary solemnly offered his life to God in a fervent prayer that the epidemic would cease. On September 17, 1866, Brother Francis Mary died from the cholera he had contracted while nursing its victims.

Immediately after Francis Mary's death, people began reporting miraculous cures at his tomb.

Pope St. John XXIII canonized him on December 9, 1962.

St. Francis Mary of Camporosso's feast day is September 17.

33

St. Francis Xavier, S.J.
April 7, 1506 – December 3, 1552

FRANCIS XAVIER WAS BORN ON April 7, 1506 to a wealthy family in Navarre, in what is now Spain.

When he was 17 years old, Francis attended the University of Paris and received his licentiate in 1528. While there, he met another Spanish nobleman named Ignatius of Loyola. Ignatius, Francis Xavier, and five other men vowed themselves to serve God as "spiritual warriors." These men were ordained priests in Venice in 1534 and became known as the Society of Jesus (Jesuits). They pledged themselves to serve God wherever they were called to do so in the world.

In 1540, Fr. Ignatius appointed Francis to join Fr. Simón Rodriguez to go to the East Indies. When Francis found Simón, he had moved to Portugal and was nursing the sick in a hospital in Lisbon. Francis promptly joined Simón in nursing the sick and teaching the patients the faith.

King John III of Portugal loved Fathers Simón and Francis, and he wanted to keep them in his country. But he agreed to let them go when the men showed him documents from the pope that appointed Francis the apostolic nuncio to the Far East.

Before Francis Xavier and his companions began their journey, the king wanted to shower them with gifts, including a servant for Francis. Francis refused most of the gifts, including the servant, saying "The best means to acquire true dignity is to wash one's own clothes and boil one's own pot, unbeholden to anyone."

On his 35th birthday, April 7 1541, Francis Xavier and his companions (including two priests) began their amazing missionary journey. Fr. Francis sailed in the flagship, and his companions sailed in another ship. This journey to Goa, a Portuguese colony in India, would last 13 months and be filled with many challenges.

On the journey, Fr. Francis found himself once again in the nursing role. He considered himself responsible for the welfare of all on board the ship, but in particular for their health care. In addition to the ship's crew, there were paying passengers, soldiers, slaves, and convicts. Francis treated them all with respect and dignity.

During this voyage, Francis celebrated Mass every Sunday and taught the Catholic faith. He also nursed the sick as best he could, even though he himself frequently suffered from seasickness. Scurvy and other illnesses plagued the journey, and Fr. Francis turned his own cabin into an infirmary to care for the sickest of all.

On May 6, 1542, the ships finally landed at Goa. He discovered that although the Portuguese had established Catholic parishes in Goa, they were treating the natives abusively.

In this new land, Fr. Francis immediately went to work nursing the sick in hospitals and prisons, and teaching the catechism to children and slaves. He celebrated Mass with lepers every Sunday and preached in the streets. He even created simple songs to teach the people basic dogmas of the faith.

After working in Goa for five months, Fr. Francis began working in other areas of India, in Japan, and a number of island nations. Though he longed to take the Christian faith to China, he was never able to do that.

Fr. Francis Xavier gave himself entirely to the people he served. He ate a simple diet of rice and water, and he slept on a floor in a hut. In every possible way he was a "missionary's missionary." In fact, he was one of the most amazing missionaries in Catholic history.

On December 3, 1552, Fr. Francis Xavier died in a Portuguese island colony off the coast of China at the age of 46. There were only four people at his funeral.

In his eleven years as a missionary in the East, Francis Xavier opened up Christian mission territories in India, Sri Lanka, Malaysia, and Japan.

Pope Gregory XV canonized Francis Xavier in 1622, and Pope Pius XI named him a patron saint of foreign missionaries. Many universities and other institutions throughout the world are named in honor of St. Francis Xavier.

St. Francis Xavier's feast day is December 3.

34

Bl. Francis Xavier Seelos, C.Ss.R.
January 11, 1819 – October 4, 1867

FRANCIS XAVIER SEELOS WAS BORN in Füssen, Bavaria on January 11, 1819. He was the sixth child born into a family that would eventually have 12 children. He was baptized on the same day at his parents' parish church of St. Mang.

Clues to Francis' eventual vocation to the priesthood were seen in childhood, when he would set up an altar at home and hold services for his little friends.

After completing his philosophy education at the University of Munich, Francis entered a diocesan seminary in 1842. One day, however, he read in a Redemptorist missionary newspaper called *Sion,* that German-speaking immigrants in the United States lacked spiritual care. Therefore, he applied to, and was accepted by, the Redemptorist Order.

Francis Xavier Seelos departed for the United States on March 17, 1843 from the port of Le Havre on the ship *Saint Nicholas* and arrived in New York City on April 20, 1843.

He served his novitiate year in Baltimore, and on May 16, 1844, he took his first vows in the Redemptorist order. On December 22, 1844, Francis was ordained a priest.

After serving at St. James Church in Baltimore for 6 months, he was sent to St. Philomena Church in Pittsburgh. This church was nicknamed "the factory church" for it was a makeshift church originally built as a factory.

Fr. Francis grew and flourished under the direction of his pastor, St. John Neumann, a Bohemian Redemptorist. Soon stories began circulating about how generous and kind Fr. Francis was to the poor, notably his love of the sick. Sometimes, for example, he would do private duty nursing for a sick child so that a mother with an exhausting job outside the home, could have a break.

Fr. Francis did all the usual duties of a parish priest— baptizing infants, witnessing weddings, visiting the sick, celebrating Reconciliation, counseling individuals and couples, and the myriad other things parish priests do. He preached to his largely immigrant congregations in English, German, and French.

People loved Fr. Francis' sermons because they were simple and highly entertaining, despite his poor English. His sermons evidenced his very deep pastoral love for the people.

Fr. Francis cared so much for the sick that often he would sleep in his clothes at night near a particularly sick person's front door, so that he could go in at a moment's notice if needed.

Though his parishioners loved him, Fr. Francis encountered anti-Catholic bigots from time to time. At various times he was brutally beaten, pelted with rocks, threatened at gunpoint, and nearly thrown overboard a ferryboat while carrying the Blessed Sacrament with him.

On March 1854, Fr. Francis became pastor of St. Alphonsus parish in Baltimore and was appointed director of students at the Redemptorist seminary.

In March 1857, Fr. Francis was sent to Annapolis as pastor of a very small parish named St. Mary and was appointed novice master for the Redemptorists. This assignment lasted only two months, and then his superiors sent him to an even smaller church in Cumberland, Maryland – Saints Peter and Paul. He also was made director of a Redemptorist seminary.

In the seminary, Fr. Francis was highly popular with the seminarians because he was very progressive for his time. He was very approachable and even playful with the students. Once, for example, he asked if he could become a member of the Laughing Society that three students had formed.

Fr. Seelos' popularity with the students made many other priests jealous of him. His peers' jealousy, however, did not make him change his joyful, Spirit-led, progressive style.

In 1865 Fr. Francis served in Detroit, and in September 1866 he was transferred to St. Mary's Church in the Irish section of New Orleans. During this time a yellow fever epidemic was devastating New Orleans. Fr. Francis nursed the sick and met their spiritual needs. But as a result of his nursing, he contacted yellow fever and died on October 4, 1867. His nursing earned him the title of "martyr to charity."

Fr. Francis Xavier Seelos was buried next to Brother Wenceslaus Neumann - St. John Neumann's brother - at St. Mary's in New Orleans.

On January 11, 2013, the Seelos Center was dedicated at Research College of Nursing at Rockhurst University in Kansas City, Missouri. This facility has classrooms, meeting spaces, nursing simulation labs, lounges, and offices, all designed to assist nursing students to one day become great nurses.

Pope St. John Paul II beatified Francis Xavier Seelos on April 9, 2000.

Blessed Francis Xavier Seelos' feast day is October 5.

35

St. Gaspar Bertoni, C.S.S.
October 9, 1777 – June 12, 1853

GASPAR BERTONI WAS BORN TO a prosperous family on October 9, 1777 in Verona, Republic of Venice.

The day after he was born, his granduncle, Fr. James Bertoni, baptized him. When his sister died, he was the only child.

Gaspar received an excellent education at home as well as in schools run by the Jesuits and a Marian congregation. When he was 11, Gaspar received his First Communion. From that time on, he became very spiritual.

When he was 18 years old, Gaspar entered a seminary. Unfortunately, during his first year of theology in 1796, the French army invaded the city where he was studying. This invasion began a 20-year period of turmoil.

Gaspar was deeply affected by the devastation around him. As a result, he joined a newly formed group called the Gospel Fraternity for the Hospitals founded by Servant of God Peter Leonardi.

In this fraternity, Gaspar began nursing the sick and wounded soldiers. While nursing, he gained insight into the lives of those he tended. Such insight would eventually help him cope with his own illness later in life.

On September 20, 1800, Gaspar was ordained a diocesan priest and assigned to a parish. Filled with the energy that all new priests have, he immersed himself in youth ministry.

In 1810 he was transferred to a new parish and entrusted by the bishop to become the spiritual director of the diocesan seminary. He loved having young people at his home for conversation and faith formation.

When Napoleon Bonaparte came into power he suppressed many religious movements, including many in the Catholic Church. This caused great turmoil and disorganization in the Church.

In 1816, after Napoleon's defeat, Fr. Gaspar founded a new religious community called the Congregation of the Sacred Stigmata of Our Lord Jesus Christ – more commonly called the Stigmatines.

The Stigmatines opened a tuition-free school and worked for the betterment of society and Church.

On May 30, 1812, Fr. Gaspar became ill with what in those days was called "military fever," most likely yellow fever. Though he recovered, he remained in poor health for the rest of his 41 years on earth.

Even from his sick bed, Gaspar practiced what would today be called psychosocial nursing and spiritual counseling. In fact, he became known "the angel of counsel." Among his many visitors was Blessed Charles Steeb.

Fr. Gaspar died on June 12, 1853.

Pope St. John Paul II canonized him on November 1, 1989.

St. Gaspar Bertoni's feast day is June 12.

36

St. Gerard Majella, C.Ss.R.
April 6, 1726 – October 16, 1755

GERARD MAJELLA WAS BORN THE youngest of five children on April 6, 1726 in Muro Lucano, Basilicata, in the south of what is now Italy.

When Gerard was twelve, his father, a tailor, died, leaving the family in poverty. Gerard's mother sent him to live with her brother so he could also learn the tailor's trade. Unfortunately, the foreman was abusive toward Gerard. Despite the abuse, Gerard kept silent. When Gerard's uncle found out, however, he fired the foreman. This incident is important, because it shows a pattern that would recur in Gerard's life, that is, being silent in the face of persecution.

After four years as a tailor apprentice, Gerard became a servant to the Bishop of Lacedonia. When the bishop died, Gerard went to work as a tailor in his own right. He gave his earnings to his mother, to the poor, and as offerings for Masses for the "poor souls in purgatory."

When he was a young man, Gerard tried to become a Capuchin Franciscan, but was turned down twice due to his frail health.

Gerard did not give up his dream to enter the Religious life in spite of rejection. In fact, one priest, about to leave town, advised Gerard's mother to lock Gerard in his room so that he would not follow. Gerard's mother did just that, but in the morning, when she unlocked Gerard's room, she found that he had gone out the window and climbed to the ground with the help of a sheet. He left her a note on the table that said, "I have gone to become a Saint."

The priest who had discouraged Gerard from entering Religious life finally gave in. Gerard's letter of introduction from the priest to the Redemptorist house said, "I am sending you a useless lay brother."

So in 1749, when Gerard was 23, the Congregation of the Most Holy Redeemer (Redemptorists) accepted him as a lay Brother. They soon discovered, however, that this "useless lay brother" could do the work of four men.

In his time in the Order, Brother Gerard served his community as a porter, tailor, sacristan, gardener, and as a nurse. And even though he was not a priest, his superiors permitted him to counsel communities of women Religious because of his gift of "reading consciences" or "reading souls." When engaged in such activity, he was what one might call a psychosocial-spiritual nurse.

Though Gerard had many different jobs, he was frequently called on to help the sick and the poor.

Gerard nursed those sick in mind, spirit and body, but was also an instrument God frequently used to perform miracles. Among his many miracles were raising a boy from the dead after the boy had fallen from a high cliff; blessing a poor farmer's crops which ridded it of mice; blessing a poor family's wheat supply, enabling the wheat to last until the next harvest; and multiplying bread on several occasions.

The miracle for which Brother Gerard is most famous, however, is his help to a young pregnant woman shortly before his death. Brother Gerard one day dropped his handkerchief. The young woman found the handkerchief and tried to return it. Gerard, however, told her to keep it for she might need it one day.

Years after Brother Gerard died, this same woman went into labor and was on the verge of losing her baby. She remembered Brother Gerard's words about keeping the handkerchief in case she needed it one day. She called for the handkerchief, and as soon as it touched her body, all pain left and all danger to the mother and baby were gone.

Though Brother Gerard was known for his amazing obedience, he was also noted for his humility, meekness, and ability to bear false witness gracefully. He demonstrated this quality when a woman accused him of improper behavior. When Brother Gerard's superior – St. Alphonsus – asked him about the accusation, Gerard simply remained silent. Only later did the woman confess she had manufactured the story.

Brother Gerard Majella died at the age of 29 on October 16, 1755 in Materdomini, Campania, Kingdom of Naples.

Pope St. Pius X canonized him on December 11, 1904.

St. Gerard Majella's feast day is October 16.

St. Gerard Majella is a patron saint of children (especially the unborn), pregnant women, mothers, falsely accused people, good confessions, lay brothers, and Muro Lucano, Italy.

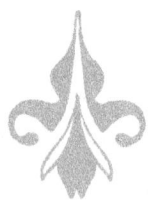

37

Bl. Gerard Meccati

c. 1174 - c. 1245

GERARD MECCATI WAS BORN AROUND 1174 in Villamagna, in the Lazio region of what is now Italy. Most of the details of his life are shrouded in mystery.

In adulthood, Gerard became a hermit. Like many hermits, he was known for his austere lifestyle and deep prayer life.

Gerard's eremitic life was fairly structured. For example, he devoted certain days of the week to praying for specific intentions. Mondays he devoted himself for praying for souls in purgatory. On Wednesdays, he prayed for the forgiveness of his sins. And on Fridays, he prayed for the conversion of the infidels. The "infidels," in the time Gerard lived, referred to Muslims.

Church historians believe that one point in his life he was a pilgrim and settled at the hospital of St. John of Jerusalem. There he worked many years nursing the sick in what was considered one of the finest hospitals of that time. In addition to nursing the sick, he also spent time welcoming pilgrims. Gerard might have been a Brother of the Order of St. John of Jerusalem, but there is no confirmation of that.

After nursing the sick for some time, he once again became a hermit.

Blessed Gerard Meccati died around 1245.

Pope Gregory XVI beatified Gerard in 1833.

Blessed Gerard Meccati's feast day is May 13.

38

Bl. Gerard Thom
c. 1040 – September 3, 1120

GERARD THOM WAS BORN SOMETIME in 1040. His early life is shrouded in mystery, but many historians believe he may have been from Italy.

Historians also believe he was a religious Brother of some kind - perhaps a Benedictine monk.

Though little is known about his early life, we do know he was famous for his love of the sick, especially those who were poor.

It was not until his adulthood that Gerard's life adventures were recorded. We know, for example, that during the First Crusade (1095-1099), Christians were expelled from Jerusalem. Gerard, who was there at the time, was permitted to stay behind and, with some other Brothers, was able to continue nursing the sick.

After the First Crusade, Gerard continued nursing the sick in a hospital. Now, in addition to caring for the everyday patients, he was now faced with caring for many wounded knights coming back from battle. One of those knights was a nobleman named Raymond du Puy, who would one day be the successor of the religious community that Gerard would one day found.

Raymond du Puy was impressed with Gerard's compassion, sensitivity, and superb nursing care. As a result, Raymond gave Gerard some land and money to expand his nursing endeavors.

Gerard made good use of the money and the land, and soon he had a thriving hospital. As his hospital grew, Gerard founded a new religious community to care for the sick and the poor. He adopted a Rule based on the Rules of St. Benedict and St. Augustine. His men wore a black habit with a white, eight-point cross on it. In 1113, Pope Paschal II established Gerard's community as a religious Order dedicated "to serving Christ through serving the sick and poor." This Order was called the Knights Hospitallers.

Brother Gerard continued nursing the sick and caring for the poor for another 24 years. The date of his death (September 3) is known but the year is uncertain (1118-1121).

The epitaph on his tomb at the Hospital of St. John reads:

"Here lies Gerard, the humblest man in the East, the slave of the poor, hospitable to strangers, meek of countenance but with a noble heart. One can see in these walls how good he was. He was provident and active. Exerting himself in all sorts of ways, he stretched forth his arms into many lands to obtain what he needed to feed his own. On the seventeenth day of the passage of the sun under the sign of Virgo (September 3, 1120), he was carried into heaven by the hands of angels."

Many groups in the Catholic Church trace their founding to Gerard include the Knights Hospitallers, the Military and Hospitaller Order of St. Lazarus of Jerusalem, the Order of the Knights of St. John of Jerusalem, and the Order of Malta.

Blessed Gerard Thom's feast day is October 13.

39

St. Gerlac

c. 1100 – c 1170

GERLAC WAS BORN AROUND 1100 in the Netherlands.

As a young man, Gerlac served as a soldier and lived a very wild, sensuous life. Some historians also believe that Gerlac was a highwayman, a person who robs people as they travel from one place to another.

He later got married. When his wife died, Gerlac experienced a profound interior conversion.

Filled with shame and remorse, Gerlac determined to do penance to make up for his previous lifestyle. Therefore, he journeyed to Rome in 1151. There, Pope Eugenius III gave him the penance of serving as a nurse in Jerusalem for seven years. Gerlac was very happy to nurse the sick in hospitals and also serve the sick and poor in the streets.

When his seven years of nursing in Jerusalem were finished, Gerlac returned to Rome and met with Pope Adrian IV. Pope Adrian tried to talk Gerlac into joining a religious community, but Gerlac decided that was not his true calling. Rather, he felt God was calling him to the eremitic lifestyle.

Gerlac, therefore, returned to the Netherlands in Houthem, his former estate, and gave away all of his possessions to the poor. He then took up residence in a hollowed-out oak tree. For food, he ate bread mixed with ashes. Each day, he would walk to the town of Maastricht to the Basilica of Saint Servatius.

Unfortunately for Gerlac, monks of a local monastery wanted him to become one of them, but he refused. Angry at his refusal, the monks went to the bishop and convinced him that Gerlac had a fortune buried in his hollowed oak hermitage. The bishop believed the monks, and cut down poor Gerlac's tree. When the bishop discovered that Gerlac was as poor as one could possibly be, he felt very guilty for his behavior. Therefore, to make up for his mistake, the bishop ordered that the workers should make planks from the oak and build a little hermitage for Gerlac.

There are many legends associated with St. Gerlac. For example, one legend says that when Gerlac had done enough penance to make up for his wild younger days, God changed the water from a local well into wine three times to show Gerlac that all was forgiven. Another legend says that St. Servatius, an Armenian missionary who died in 384 A.D., came back to life to anoint Gerlac before he died.

St. Gerlac is a patron saint of domestic animals, and in religious art, he is often shown as a hermit with a donkey near him, or as a hermit in a hollowed-out tree.

St. Gerlac's feast day is January 5.

40

St. Henry Morse, S.J.
1595 – February 1, 1645

HENRY MORSE WAS BORN SOMETIME in 1595 in Brome, Suffolk, England to a Protestant family.

While studying at the English College in Rome, Henry became a Catholic Christian on June 5, 1614. Later, he was ordained a priest in Rome.

He left for the English Catholic missions in September of 1620, a time when England had adopted strong anti-Catholic laws. As a Catholic priest, he was caught and sentenced to three years in York Castle.

While in the castle, Henry developed a close friendship with a fellow prisoner, Jesuit Fr. John Robinson. While in the prison, Henry made his novitiate in the Society of Jesus (Jesuits) and, as his three-year sentence drew to an end, he made his simple vows.

After he was released from prison, Fr. Henry was banished from England and went to Flanders. There, he served English mercenary soldiers fighting for Spain.

In 1633, Fr. Henry returned to England under the name "Cuthbert Claxton" and continued his priestly ministry in London.

In 1636-1637, while he was still in London, a plague epidemic struck the city. With no thought to his own well-being, Fr. Henry began nursing the sick. In addition to nursing, he also helped gather material goods for over 400 families. As a result of Fr. Henry's compassionate nursing of mind, body, and spirit, over 100 Protestant families returned to the Catholic Church.

In 1641, the English government ordered all Catholic priests to leave England. Once again, Henry found his way to Flanders. Two years later, however, he made his way back to England, again worked as a priest, and again was arrested and sentenced to death.

Fr. Henry Morse was executed on February 1, 1645. In his honor, French, Spanish, and Portuguese ambassadors were present.

Pope Paul VI canonized Henry on October 25, 1970 as one of the 40 Martyrs of England and Wales.

St. Henry Morse's feast day is February 1, and additionally his life is celebrated on October 25, the feast of the Forty Martyrs of England and Wales.

41

Fr. Henri Nouwen
January 24, 1932 – September 21, 1996

HENRI JOZEF MACHIEL NOUWEN WAS born in Nijkerk, the Netherlands, on January 24, 1932. Henri was the eldest of four children. His father was a tax attorney, and his mother was a bookkeeper in her family's business.

As a young man, Henri studied at Aloysius College in The Hague and then spent a year at the minor seminary in Apeldoorn. Following Apeldoorn, Henri studied six years at the major seminary in Rijsenburg.

Henri was ordained a Catholic priest for the Archdiocese of Utrecht on July 21, 1957. Because he had a great desire to learn more about himself and those he counseled, he asked for permission to study psychology instead of theology, and the archdiocesan officials granted his request. From 1957 to 1964 he studied at Catholic University in Nijmegen. For his doctoral thesis, he focused on Anton Boisen, an American Protestant minister who founded the clinical pastoral education (CPE) movement. Unfortunately, his dissertation was not accepted, and he never did receive his Ph.D. Rather, he received what was called a *doctorandus* degree; today, we would call it an "ABD" or "all-but-dissertation."

After receiving his *doctorandus*, Fr. Henri studied as a Fellow in the Religion and Psychiatry Program at the Menninger Clinic in Topeka, Kansas based on the advice of psychologist Dr. Gordon Allport. Fr. Henri also did his CPE training at Topeka State Hospital and graduated from the Menninger

Foundation's training program in theology and psychiatric theory on June 19, 1965.

The 1960s were a tumultuous and exciting period of American history, and Fr. Henri wanted to be part of it. Excited by the civil rights movement, he participated in the Selma to Montgomery marches.

From 1966 to 1968, he was a visiting professor at the University of Notre Dame in Indiana, and from 1968 to 1970 he taught psychology and spirituality at the Catholic Theological Institute in Utrecht while also serving at the Amsterdam Joint Pastoral Institute.

From 1971 to 1981, Fr. Henri was a professor of pastoral theology at Yale Divinity School and was a regular contributor to the *National Catholic Reporter*. While at Yale, Fr. Henri took various sabbaticals and did much writing during these periods. For example, he was a Fellow at the Collegeville Institute for Ecumenical and Cultural Research at St. John's Abbey, and in 1978 he was a scholar-in-residence at the Pontifical North American College in Rome.

His seven-month visit to the Trappist Abbey of the Genesee in New York led to his book, *Genesee Diary: Report from a Trappist Monastery*. After leaving Yale he traveled to Bolivia and Peru, from which trip came his book, *Gracias: A Latin American Journal*.

Although Fr. Henri Nouwen published 39 books and wrote hundreds of articles before his death, his most famous book is *The Wounded Healer*. This book discusses the importance of suffering in the life of the caregiver, for if the caregiver does not know suffering, he or she cannot fully appreciate the suffering of one's patients.

It was not until the last chapter of his life, however, that Fr. Henri Nouwen discovered nursing as a source of joy and fulfillment.

Fr. Henri's journey into nursing began in 1985 when he met Jean Vanier, a Canadian Catholic philosopher, theologian, and humanitarian who in 1964 founded L'Arche, an international federation of communities for people with developmental disabilities and those who assist them.

Eventually, Fr. Henri found himself at L'Arche Daybreak community in Richmond Hill, a city near Toronto. There, Fr. Henri spent the last ten years of his life. While at Daybreak, Fr. Henri was paired with a young man with severe developmental disabilities named Adam Arnett.

Fr. Henri became Adam's primary caretaker. As such, he was responsible for total patient care – meeting the biophysical and psychosocial aspects of nursing care. Though he was not a professional nurse, Fr. Henri learned on the job how to do the basics. From this experience, Fr. Henri learned deeply how to see Christ in every human being, and he learned what it meant to serve others completely. From his experience, Fr. Henri Nouwen wrote his final book – *Adam: God's Beloved*.

Fr. Henri Nouwen died on September 21, 1996 in Hilversum, Netherlands, at the age of 64. A number of awards and schools have been named after him, and books continue to be written about his remarkably productive and exciting life.

42

Bl. Hugolino of Magalotti, O.S.F.
Died December 11, 1373

VERY LITTLE IS KNOWN ABOUT Hugolino of Magalotti, but it is believed he was born in the early fourteenth century in Camerino, Papal States.

As a young man, he lost his parents and received an inheritance, which he promptly gave away to the poor.

He then became a member of the Third Order of St. Francis and went to live as a hermit. He spent his days praying, doing penance, and engaging in various manual labors. Soon people began to learn about Hugolino's holiness. And, just as moths are attracted to light, people are attracted to people who radiate goodness.

The sick, especially, were attracted to Hugolino. Not only did Hugolino nurse the sick, he often cured them. In fact, many miracles were attributed to Hugolino both during his life and after his death.

Hugolino died on December 11, 1373. At his funeral, a large number of people came to honor him.

Hugolino became a "Blessed" of the Catholic Church in 1856.

Blessed Hugolino's feast day is December 11.

43

St. Ivo of Brittany
October 17, 1235 – May 19, 1303

Ivo of Brittany, also known as Ivo of Kermartin, was born on October 17, 1235 in a manor near Tréguier in Brittany, now part of France.

As a young man, Ivo studied canon law and theology at the University of Paris for ten years, and civil law for three years at Orleans.

While other students lived the typical party lifestyle, Ivo studied hard. In his free time, he loved to pray and to visit the sick.

In 1262, Ivo returned to Brittany and was appointed a judge in the church courts of the Diocese of Rennes. Soon, however, the bishop of Tréguier called Ivo to serve in the same position in his home diocese.

Ivo became known for his remarkable fairness and impartiality, and became known as a champion of the poor, giving them special attention. Often he tried to persuade litigants to settle their differences out of court. His solid reputation became so great, in fact, that it gave rise to a verse that people of the time used to say: "St. Ivo was a Breton, a lawyer not a robber; astonishing in people's eyes."

In 1284, when he was about 49 years old, Ivo was ordained a priest and assigned to lead the parish of Tredrez. In 1287, Fr. Ivo resigned from his legal offices and devoted himself full-time to his parish.

After a few years, Fr. Ivo was sent to a more prestigious parish in Lovannec. There he built a hospital. Not only did he spend time nursing the sick, he also gave special attention to vagrants. Fr. Ivo not only nursed the minds and bodies of his patients, he also worked hard for their spiritual well being.

Fr. Ivo became ill during Lent in 1303. On May 10, 1303, Fr. Ivo celebrated his last Mass. At that Mass, he had to have physical assistance, and only with great effort could he preach a homily. Fr. Ivo died on May 19, 1303.

Pope Clement VI canonized Ivo in June of 1347.

St. Ivo's feast day is May 19. St. Ivo is a patron saint of Brittany, lawyers, judges, and abandoned children.

44

Bl. James of Bitetto, O.F.M.
c. 1400 - 1485

JAMES OF BITETTO, SOMETIMES KNOWN as "James the Slav" or "James the Illyrian," was born around 1400 in Zara, Dalmatia.

As with many holy people of that time, few details of his life were recorded.

We do know that James became a lay brother in the Franciscan house in his hometown when he was twenty years old.

In 1438, Brother James went with his provincial to Bitetto, a small town in the southern part of the Italian peninsula. There, James served in many houses of the Order in the region, and finally in Bitetto itself. Though he worked as a cook and other jobs, his special job in the Bitetto house was that of begging for alms for the house.

In addition to becoming known for his great holiness, humility, self-denial, and prayer life, he was seen going into ecstasy at times.

Brother James, however, also distinguished himself as a nurse during the plague that came to Bitetto in 1482.

Brother James died in 1485, and Pope Clement XI beatified him in December of 1700.

Blessed James of Bitetto's feast day is April 27.

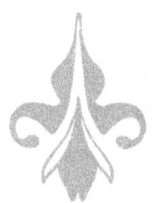

45

Bl. James of Lodi, O.S.F.
1364 – April 18, 1404

JAMES OF LODI, ALSO KNOWN as James of Oldo, was born in 1364 to a wealthy family in Lodi, a town near Milan.

When he grew up, he married Caterina Bocconi who, like him, enjoyed the finer things of life. The couple had three children. Life was good for this young family until plague came to Lodi.

When the plague came to their town, the couple fled with their children to the countryside to avoid becoming sick. Unfortunately, however, two of their daughters had already caught the plague and soon died.

When the couple returned to Lodi, James experienced a total conversion. He realized what folly it was to build up treasures on earth, when he should be building up treasure in heaven. James began spending much time in his parish church and doing penance for his sins.

James also did private-duty nursing for a sick priest who had taught him Latin.

James and his wife became members of the Third Order of St. Francis and gave up sexual relations with each other.

After Caterina died, James was ordained a priest in 1397. He turned his house into a chapel and opened it up to others. Many small groups of people came there to pray and to seek mutual support.

Fr. James threw himself into nursing the sick, especially prisoners of war. While nursing the sick, however, he caught an infectious disease and died on April 18, 1404.

Fr. James was buried in St. Julian Church, which he and his wife had founded.

Soon, people began reporting miracles that had occurred at his tomb. In fact, so many people came to honor him, that his body was transferred to a larger church and then, in 1789, to the cathedral. James has been honored as a Blessed since 1933.

Blessed James of Lodi's feast day is April 18.

46

Bl. Jeremy of Valacchia, O.F.M. Cap.
June 7, 1556 – February 26, 1625

JOHN KOSTISTIK WAS BORN ON June 7, 1556 in Zazo in Valacchia, Romania. John's family had a successful farm, and the family was known for giving what they could to the poor. John's mother, for example, baked bread from extra grain for those who were hungry, and John and his grandfather chopped wood for the poor.

When he was 18 years old, John left Romania, at his mother's prompting, to seek a life for himself in the southern part of Italy.

John's first four years in the south did not go very well for the young man, so someone told him he should go to Naples to try his luck there.

In Naples, John joined the Capuchin Franciscan Order. He was given the habit and name of Jeremy in 1578. One year later, he made his profession.

After making his profession, Brother Jeremy began nursing the sick. This he did until he died. Although he cared for the sick in various friaries, in 1585 he was assigned to the infirmary of the Monastery of St. Ephrem the Old in Naples. There, he nursed the sick not only of his religious community, but also of the general population.

Brother Jeremy became known throughout Naples for his compassion for the suffering and holiness. For Jeremy, his patients were simply part of the "suffering Jesus." Often, Jeremy would be found praying in the middle of the night in spite of having put in full days of nursing.

Brother Jeremy also developed an herbal preparation to cover the stench of the rotting flesh of lepers for whom he cared. Soon, people began talking about miraculous cures that came from Jeremy's nursing care and prayers.

In addition to basic biophysical nursing, Brother Jeremy was an excellent nurse of the mentally ill. Once, for example, he became the private-duty nurse of a friar who would become so violent that he drove everyone else away. He cared for that friar for five years. He called this nursing experience his "recreation."

Jeremy also developed a reputation for taking Franciscan poverty above and beyond what was reasonably expected. He spent 35 years, for example, wearing the same habit, and he would often give his food away to those in need.

On February 26, 1625, a member of the Naples royal court, John Avales, was gravely ill and asked Brother Jeremy to make a nursing visit. Jeremy, now 69 years old, did not hesitate. Unfortunately, the place he had to walk was seven miles away. Nevertheless, Jeremy made the journey on a cold, wet winter's night. This journey brought on double pneumonia from which he never recovered.

Brother Jeremy died on February 26, 1625.

Pope St. John Paul II beatified Jeremy on October 30, 1983, the first Romanian ever to be beatified.

Blessed Jeremy's feast day is October 30.

47

St. Jerome Emiliani, C.R.S.
1481 – February 8, 1537

JEROME EMILIANI WAS BORN IN Venice sometime in 1481. When he was only five years old, his father died.

At the age of 15, Jerome ran away from home to join the army of the City-State of Venice. Unfortunately, in one battle, he was captured and chained in a dungeon.

While in prison, Jerome began thinking about his life and what he wanted to do with it. Although he did not have much use for religion before his imprisonment, he now turned to God in a special way. He also made a vow to the Virgin Mary. Jerome was able to miraculously escape, which he attributed to Mary's intervention. As a result of his escape, he made his way to Treviso where he hung up his chains in the church. Eventually, he became mayor of the town.

Jerome did not stay long in Treviso. Instead, he returned to Venice to oversee the education of his nephews and study for the priesthood. In 1518, Jerome was ordained a priest.

At that time, there was not only a famine causing much suffering in the area, but also plague was devastating the population. Fr. Jerome, with great zeal and passion, threw himself into nursing the sick and feeding the hungry at his own expense. He also developed a special love for orphans and abandoned children and rented a house for them. There, he would teach them catechism and made sure they had food and clothes. During this time, Fr. Jerome caught the plague while nursing the sick, but he recovered.

In 1531, Fr. Jerome expanded his work to other cities, founding orphanages, hospitals, and a home for former prostitutes.

With two other priests, Jerome founded a new religious congregation called the Clerks Regular of Somasca – or Somaschi for short. The main work of this new Order was to care for orphans.

Fr. Jerome died on February 8, 1537 from an infectious disease that he caught while nursing the sick.

Pope Clement XIII canonized Jerome on October 12, 1767. Pope Pius XI declared him to be a patron saint of orphans and abandoned children in 1928.

St. Jerome Emiliani's feast day is February 8.

48

St. John Baptist de Rossi
February 22, 1698 – May 23, 1764

JOHN BAPTIST DE ROSSI WAS born on February 22, 1698 in Voltaggio near Genoa.

When he was just ten years old, a Genoese noble and his wife asked John's family if they could informally adopt him and provide him a good education. John's parents agreed.

When he was only 13 years old, John entered the Roman College. Unfortunately, he was not a prudent teenager: he studied too hard, and was into great mortification of the body, a form of spirituality common in that day. As a result of his severe lifestyle and epilepsy, he suffered a breakdown.

John recovered and was ordained a priest in 1721. For 40 years, he served as simple assistant parish priest in Rome. His love of asceticism, which had shown itself in his younger years, remained with him in adulthood. As a priest, he lived in an attic in severe poverty.

Though he was a poor and simple man, Fr. John touched the lives of thousands of people through his sensitivity and compassion.

Fr. John not only had a great devotion to the sick, he also loved to help the underdogs of society – prostitutes, prisoners, the homeless, and others.

Fr. John loved nursing the sick, and that is probably what he is most famous for. According to those who knew him, there was no task that he considered to be beneath him as a nurse. He did all he could to relieve human suffering through his psychosocial and biophysical nursing practice.

Through his nursing, John was able to demonstrate humility and compassion that melted hardened hearts. Once, for example, he ministered to a young man who was dying from syphilis. The young man rejected Fr. John's every effort to help the young man get right with the Lord. Then, one day, Fr. John emptied the young man's bedpan. This simple act so amazed the young man, that he made a good Confession before he died.

In addition to nursing the sick during the day, Fr. John could often be seen in the city at night, ministering to street people – beggars, the homeless, prostitutes, and others. Many priests were amazed at how effective Fr. John was as a confessor.

Fr. John was not shy in giving advice to fellow priests, advice that showed the pastoral sensitivity of a priest and a nurse. For example, to priests who avoided hospital ministry, Fr. John said, "Many of us shrink from going to the hospitals from fear of infection or from the sights and smells that await us there. Courage! We are not in the world to follow our own will and pleasure, but to imitate the Lord!"

And again, he cautioned priests to be sensitive to the poor of their parishes when he advised, "The poor come to church tired and distracted by their daily troubles. If you preach a long sermon they can't follow you. Give them one idea that they can take home, not half a dozen, or one will drive out the other, and they will remember none."

Fr. John wore himself out nursing the sick and caring for the outcasts of society. He suffered a stroke in 1763 and a year later he died on May 23, 1764.

Following his death, many miraculous cures were attributed to his intercession.

Pope Leo XIII canonized Fr. John on December 8, 1881.

St. John Baptist de Rossi's feast day is May 23.

49

St. John Bosco, S.D.B.
August 16, 1815 – January 31, 1888

JOHN BOSCO WAS BORN ON August 16, 1815 in hillside hamlets of Becchi, in the Piedmont region of what is now Italy, the youngest of three boys. His parents worked as farmhands in the area.

When John was only nine years old, he had a vivid dream. In the dream, he was in a field of rowdy young boys who were cursing and misbehaving. He jumped into the crowd to tame them with fists and shouting. Suddenly, however, a figure appeared to John and put him in charge of the boys. The figure told John that he should lead the boys not with anger and violence, but with gentleness and kindness. The apparition also told John that this would be his life's work.

John's older brothers made fun of him when he told them about his dreams. One brother was so harsh toward John, in fact, that John ran away from home and became a shepherd.

As a youth, John had great abilities as a juggler, magician and acrobat. With these gifts, he put on shows that attracted many youth as well as adults. Before and after his performances, he would lead the crowds in prayer.

When John was around 15, a holy priest encouraged him to enter a seminary. Because he was so poor, his friends had to take up collections to buy the clothes, books and other things he needed for the seminary.

As a young priest, Fr. John was first assigned as chaplain of a girls' boarding school, but he also visited prisons, taught catechism, and helped out in parishes. While visiting prisons, he saw young boys treated terribly. And in his ministry, he began to attract young orphan boys. He eventually enlisted his mother, "Mama Margherita," to help him take care of orphans.

Fr. John and his orphan boys were evicted from one place after another because the exuberant boys were often too noisy for the neighborhoods. When he would be thrown out of one place, he would simply find another.

In time, Fr. John attracted other men to his work, and thus began a new religious order. Because Fr. John very much admired St. Francis de Sales, his new congregation became known as the Salesian Fathers. Later, he founded the Daughters of Mary Help of Christians. This was an order for religious Sisters to do the same work for girls that Fr. John was doing for boys. Finally, he founded a group called the "Salesian Cooperators," lay people who were interested in helping him. He also published a Salesian bulletin that even today is published in many languages.

Fr. John set up schools for his boys to learn trades such as shoemaking, tailoring, bookbinding, and others. Needless to say, he also made sure every child had a safe place to live. Fr. John gave his entire life to his boys, and nothing was too good for them – especially his total devotion, love, and selflessness. In fact, Fr. John Bosco once wrote this:

> "I have promised God that until my last breath I shall have lived for my poor young people. I study for you, I work for you, I am also ready to give my life for you. Take note that whatever I am, I have been so entirely for you, day and night, morning and evening, at every moment."

Fr. John Bosco was also a leader in nursing the sick during a cholera epidemic in Turin in 1854. Recovering himself from a hemorrhage, Fr. John did not hesitate to throw himself into nursing while most of the population refused out of fear. He not only nursed the sick, but also enlisted all his boys to help him. He told the boys that as long as they trusted in God's grace and committed no mortal sins, they would not become infected. So the boys jumped in to help, carrying the sick to hospitals and the dead to mortuaries. By the time the epidemic ended, over 1,400 people had died. Not one of Fr. John's boys became infected.

We should not be surprised that Fr. John and boys were protected from cholera, for even before the epidemic, Fr. John Bosco had already gained a reputation as a miracle worker. His nursing work in the cholera epidemic, and the safe delivery of his boys, simply increased his miracle-worker reputation among the populace.

Today, Salesians are found all over the world serving poor boys and girls and leading them to a better life.

Fr. John Bosco died on January 31, 1888.

Pope Pius XI canonized him on April 1, 1934.

St. John Bosco's feast day is January 31. St. John Bosco is a patron saint of editors, publishers, schoolchildren, young people, magicians, and juvenile delinquents.

50

St. John Calabria, P.S.D.P.
October 8, 1873 – December 4, 1954

JOHN CALABRIA WAS BORN ON October 8, 1873 in Verona, Italy, youngest of seven brothers. His family was poor. So when his father died when John was in the fourth grade, John had to find work as an apprentice.

Fortunately for John, a priest helped him obtain enough of an education to be accepted into a seminary high school.

When war came, John found himself in the military. He found, however, that he had no taste for war. Therefore, he volunteered to nurse typhus patients in a military hospital. In those days, that was very dangerous work, for it was easy to become infected.

After the war, John returned to the seminary to study to become a priest. One night, while still a seminarian, John found an abandoned baby and took it home with him. This event led John to a lifelong passion for helping abandoned children and other outcasts of society.

In August of 1901, John was ordained a diocesan priest and assigned as the curate of St. Stephen parish, and confessor of the local seminary. In 1907, he was appointed rector of San Benedetto del Monte, where he nursed sick soldiers and tried to help them in any way he could.

On November 26, 1907, Fr. John founded the "Congregation of the Poor Servants of Divine Providence" which was approved by the pope on April 25, 1949. This congregation nursed the sick and elderly, and served the poor, abandoned, and outcasts of society.

Fr. John Calabria died on December 4, 1954 at the age of 81. Pope St. John Paul II canonized him on April 18, 1999. St. John Calabria's feast day is December 4.

51

Bl. John Colombini
1305 – July 31, 1367

JOHN COLOMBINI WAS BORN IN the Republic of Siena in 1305.

When he grew up, he got married, had a daughter, and became a successful businessman and senator. He threw himself into making money and getting ahead in the material world.

When he was about 50 years old, however, John became enchanted with religion. Specifically, he was touched by the life of St. Mary of Egypt in a book of the saints that his wife had given him.

Soon John began to give away large sums of money to the poor and spent several hours a day in church praying. He also devoted himself to nursing the sick and caring for the poor. In fact, he took sick people into his house, so that soon it became more like a hospital than a home. This was all too much for his long-suffering wife. So, John made financial provisions for her and their daughter and began nursing full-time in the city's hospitals.

He, and a like-minded former merchant, Francesco di Mino de' Vincent, joined forces. Soon, other men were attracted to John and Francesco and joined them in their care of the sick. Unfortunately, the Siena city fathers became alarmed at the success of this unofficial religious community and banished them from Siena.

So John left Siena with some of his followers and moved to other cities and villages. In the city of Viterbo, they became known as Gesuati – or Jesuats (not to be confused with Jesuits) – because of their devotion to the

Holy Name of Jesus and their frequent cry of "Praise be to Jesus Christ!" The city of Siena eventually welcomed John and his followers when an epidemic of bubonic plague broke out, rendering the city desperately in need of the nursing and burial services of the brothers.

When Pope Urban V passed through the area in 1367, he received John and his companions and recognized them as a new religious community called "Apostolic Clerics of St. Jerome."

This group was to be composed of lay brothers who led a life of great austerity and devoted themselves to nursing the sick and burying the dead. John's cousin, Blessed Catherine Colombini, formed a branch of cloistered nuns.

A few days after his community had received papal approval, Brother John died on July 31, 1367 as his fellow brothers were taking him back to Siena.

His congregation flourished until 1688, and the Sisters of the Visitation of Mary continued until 1872.

Pope Gregory XIII beatified John.

Blessed John Colombini's feast day is July 31.

52

St. John of the Cross, O.C.D.
1542 – December 14, 1591

JOHN WAS BORN SOMETIME IN 1542 in the town of Fontiveros near Ávila, Spain. His father, Gonzalo, was an accountant to rich silk merchant relatives. However, when Gonzalo married Catarina, a woman the relatives considered beneath their social class, they rejected Gonzalo. Gonzalo, forced to work as a weaver, died when John was only three years old.

When John was around nine, his mother sent him to an orphanage in Medina del Campo to study. There he received food and clothing, and learned to read and write. He also served as an apprentice to a carpenter, wood sculptor, and printer. Unfortunately, he discovered he had no aptitude for any of these trades.

When he was fourteen years old, he landed himself a job in the *Hospital de las Bubas*, a hospital that primarily treated people with venereal diseases. In this setting, John developed a great love for the sick and the poor, and served as what we would call today a nursing assistant. There were no tasks that he considered too menial or unpleasant to undertake. He not only washed and bandaged patients, but he sang popular songs to them and made them laugh. He found he loved to care for all people, and he was very good at it.

After three or four years, the administrator of the *Hospital de las Bubas* was so impressed with John that he offered to send him to the Jesuit College. The administrator also promised John that if he were to become a priest one day, he could return to the hospital as a chaplain.

Though John loved the sick and had a great affinity toward nursing, God had other plans for John. Instead of nursing as his vocation, John was destined to become a great mystic, mystical writer, and reformer.

In 1567, John was ordained a priest in the Carmelite order. When he went home to Medina to celebrate his first Mass of Thanksgiving at his mother's church, the prior of the Carmelite house arranged him to meet a Carmelite Sister named Teresa of Avila.

John and Teresa became very close friends, and they both discovered that they longed for a form of the Carmelite Rule more primitive or severe than what was then practiced. Together, they engaged on an amazing journey to reform the Order. Eventually, their efforts resulted in formation of the Discalced (Barefoot) Carmelites.

Fr. John and Sister Teresa both suffered terribly through the years as they sought to reform Carmel. Through these years, both of them wrote very inspirational mystical writings, which have long been revered as some of the most insightful and profound spiritual documents of all time.

Fr. John of the Cross, as he came to be known, is most famous for two mystical works: *Ascent of Mount Carmel* and *Dark Night of the Soul*.

By 1581, at the First General Chapter of the Discalced Carmelites, the Order had grown to 22 houses of men and women – 300 friars and 200 nuns.

Fr. John of the Cross died on December 14, 1591 in Úbeda, Jaén, Spain.

Pope Benedict XIII canonized John on December 27, 1726.

St. John of the Cross' feast day is December 14.

St. John of the Cross is honored as a Doctor (teacher) of the Church and is a patron saint of the contemplative life, contemplatives, mystics, mystical theology, and Spanish poets.

53

St. John Eudes, C.J.M.
November 14, 1601 – August 19, 1680

JOHN EUDES WAS BORN ON November 14, 1601 in Normandy.

As a young man, he studied with the Jesuits at Caen and joined the Oratorian Fathers on March 25, 1623. He was ordained a priest on December 20, 1625.

Immediately after ordination to the priesthood, John became ill and was bedridden for an entire year. His recovery was slow, and for two years he could only pray, read, and rest.

Just as he was well enough to get around again, plague struck near the village where he was living. He immediately asked for permission to nurse the sick and minister to their spiritual needs.

When the plague disappeared in November of 1627, Fr. John went to Caen where he exercised his priesthood as a confessor, spiritual director, and preacher. In 1630, however, plague struck Caen. Once again, Fr. John began nursing the sick. Because he understood the nature of contagion, he lived in a huge wine cask in the middle of a field during the plague, wanting not to contaminate his fellow priests or anyone else. Benedictine nuns made sure he had enough food to get by.

When he was around 32 years old, Fr. John became a parish missionary. He not only conducted many missions, but also started many religious communities to serve the needs of people whom he thought were not adequately served. For example, he founded, with Madeleine Lamy, the Sisters of Our

Lady of Charity of the Refuge in 1641. From this congregation came the Sisters of the Good Shepherd two centuries later.

John also severed his relationship with the Oratorians and founded the Congregation of Jesus and Mary, commonly called the Eudists, for the purpose of educating priests and giving parish missions.

Fr. John Eudes accomplished much in his life. When examining his life, it seems that his three-year period of illness and recovery was the time when his call to pastoral action was taking seed and growth. Then, when he was finally well, the seeds exploded in a flurry of amazing growth.

Fr. John Eudes died in Caen on August 19, 1680.

Pope Pius IX canonized him on May 31, 1925.

St. John Eudes' feast day is April 19.

54

St. John of God, O.H.
March 8, 1495 – March 8, 1550

JOHN WAS BORN ON MARCH 8, 1495 in Montemor-o-Novo, Évora, Portugal.

From the time he was a little boy, John was incredibly impulsive in his behavior when he thought God wanted him to do something. For example, when he was eight years old, he ran away from home to follow a priest who preached about exciting new worlds opening up. He never saw his parents again.

In the next years, he worked as a mountain shepherd until he was twenty-seven years old, and he then decided to become a soldier for Spain. As a soldier, he led a wild life of drinking, gambling, and pillaging like his fellow soldiers.

As a grown man, John was very susceptible to religious preachers, just as he had been as an eight-year-old child. Often he would act impulsively and imprudently in his quest for doing what he imagined to be God's will for him. One time, for example, after hearing Blessed John of Ávila speak about repentance, John was so overcome by his sins that he dashed through the town tearing off his clothes and crying. His behavior became so bizarre that he was sent to a mental hospital, where he was regularly tied down and whipped daily. He gave up his madness, however, at the intervention of Blessed John of Ávila.

John of God, as he came to be known, served the Lord as a seller of religious books and goods. But what John is most noted for is his care for the sick and poor as a nurse and nursing administrator. Eventually he gathered like-minded men around him who also devoted their lives to nursing the sick and poor. This group became known as the Brothers Hospitallers.

A little hospital, which John founded, once caught fire. As it was burning to the ground, John ran into it and saved all the patients, while others of the town stood around watching. He then raced back into the building throwing mattresses and other needed items out the window to save them. John then used an axe to separate the burning part of the building from that which was not burning.

John of God died on his 55th birthday, March 8, 1550, in Granada.

Pope Alexander VIII canonized him on October 16, 1690.

As a result of his intriguing life, St. John of God is a patron saint of nurses, nursing administrators, booksellers, firefighters, hospitals, heart patients, the sick (including the mentally ill), and the dying.

St. John of God's feast day is March 8.

55

St. John Grande-Román, O.H.
March 6, 1546 – June 3, 1600

JOHN GRANDE-ROMÁN WAS BORN ON March 6, 1546 in Carmona, Seville. Like other Catholic Christians of his time, he had close ties to the Church from his birth. He was baptized the day after he was born, and he was active in his parish choir from the ages of seven to twelve.

As a young man, John learned to be a weaver and a cloth-maker in Seville. For reasons that are not known, he underwent a spiritual crisis at the age of 17 and decided to spend some time at the Hermitage of St. Olalla.

While on retreat there, John decided to leave his occupation and dedicate himself to God. He got rid of his regular clothing and substituted a habit made of sackcloth. He renounced marriage and began calling himself *Juan Pecador* – "John the Sinner."

One day, John encountered a pair of sickly poor people on the side of the road and carried them to his hut. There, he nursed them and begged alms for them. It was not long before John began to notice others who could use his nursing and related skills, skills that would likely go to waste if he continued living as a hermit.

As a result of his encounter with those in need, John went to Jerez de la Frontera and began in earnest to nurse the sick. He especially loved caring for the sick and downtrodden in the local prison. John firmly believed that there was no human being who was too far from God's reach.

After a while, John began nursing in a local hospital. He discovered, however, that his loving passion and detailed attention to nursing the sick made officials jealous of him. This jealousy undoubtedly stemmed from the poor quality of their nursing care. As a result, they often tried to obstruct John's nursing care and to insult him.

In addition to nursing the sick, John also tried to assist street people who needed help. It was not unusual for him to go begging for food and clothing for the poor and even to obtain dowries for poor young women wanting to get married.

Because of his great devotion, a rich couple gave him funds to open his own hospital in Jerez. It was not long before this hospital became famous for its excellent care.

In 1547, an epidemic broke out in his city, and John was busier than ever nursing the sick.

He soon learned about a hospital in Granada founded by the Hospitallers of St. John of God (discussed elsewhere in this book). After visiting that hospital, John adopted the rules of the Order to his own hospital. Soon other young men came to his hospital to nurse the sick, and they became Hospitallers themselves.

Because of his great success in nursing and administration, the Cardinal-Archbishop of Seville, Rodrigo de Castro, asked John to consolidate the hospitals in the area. John did this successfully though this was a difficult and sensitive task.

When the plague came to his area, John contracted it while nursing the sick. He died on June 3, 1600.

Pope St. John Paul II canonized John on June 6, 1996.

St. John Grande-Román's feast day is June 3.

56

St. John Leonardi, O.M.D.
1541 – October 9, 1609

JOHN WAS BORN SOMETIME IN 1541 in Lucca, Tuscany. At that time, Lucca was a city-state in what is now Italy.

As a young person, he worked for a pharmacist and joined a religious confraternity before studying to become a priest.

John was ordained around 1572. As a young priest, he spent much time in his early priesthood serving patients in hospitals and people in prison in Lucca. Before long, young laymen gathered around him to help him in his work. This group lived together in community, sharing not only their ministry, but also praying together.

John was also very interested in ensuring that Catholic doctrine was being correctly taught, and that people had a good understanding of the teachings of the Council of Trent (1545-1563). In Lucca, there were preachers whose teaching on various Catholic dogmas was not orthodox. Therefore, the bishop of Lucca gave Fr. John the task of preaching in all the parishes of Lucca.

In 1574, Fr. John formally recognized his group of lay helpers as a religious community. Fr. John envisioned a community dedicated to Christian education of the people, reform of the Catholic clergy, and such works of mercy as nursing the sick.

For reasons that are unclear, Fr. John's vision met violent opposition from powerful families. Some of the opposition might have arisen because some of the un-orthodox Catholic preachers were members of powerful families of

Lucca, and some of it may have been because many priests did not want clerical reformation. Whatever the cause, Fr. John and his group were banned from Lucca, and he needed special papal protection even to visit the city.

In 1583, the bishop of Lucca, with Pope Gregory XIII's approval, officially recognized Fr. John's group. St. Philip Neri, a contemporary of John, gave the group some land, and St. Joseph Calasanz helped the group build up a good reputation throughout Italy. In 1595, Pope Clement VIII recognized Fr. John's group as a religious Congregation. (Both St. Philip Neri and St. Joseph Calasanz are other Saintly Men of Nursing in this book.) Fr. John's Order was called the Clerks Regular of the Mother of God.

Fr. John was also a founder of a special seminary for the education of foreign missionaries, later to be associated with the Society for the Propagation of the Faith. John also was responsible for reforming certain Benedictine monasteries. Fr. John also had great love for Forty Hours Devotion and frequently partook of Communion.

In 1609, Fr. John devoted himself to nursing the sick during a plague epidemic, and in October of that year, he died from the plague.

Pope Pius XI canonized John Leonardi in 1938.

St. John Leonardi's feast day is October 9.

57

Bl. John Pelingotto, O.S.F.
1240 – June 1, 1304

JOHN PELINGOTTO WAS BORN SOMETIME in 1240 in Urbino, a city in the central part of the Italian peninsula, to a prosperous merchant and his wife in the town. Though his family was able to provide him with a very comfortable life, from a very young age John had no desire for things of the material world.

As a young man, he very much wanted to leave home to become a hermit, but he stayed when his parents opposed his plan.

So John became a merchant like his father, but he was absolutely no good at it. Instead of trying to make money, he was always inclined to give away merchandise to the poor.

In addition to being a poor businessman, John lacked the social skills needed to be successful in business. In fact, when he was not working, he lived in his parents' house as a recluse.

Because of his dismal performance in the world of business, John's father reluctantly gave his blessing for John to give up his career and find something in life that would fulfill him.

John immediately decided to devote his life to nursing the sick and caring for the poor. He nursed the sick with sensitivity and compassion, but sometimes he endangered his own well-being while doing so. For example, he would often give away his food to his patients and go hungry.

Although John seems to have great success in caring for his patients and serving the poor very well, he may have been mentally ill. For example, one time, on Palm Sunday, he showed up in the cathedral with a rope tied around his neck holding a sign that said he was the worst of criminals. He also frequently gave away all his clothes, even in cold weather, and then walked around in scraps of burlap bags. Once he went into a catatonic state for several hours in the cathedral.

Fortunately, John eventually joined the Third Order of St. Francis. With the help of the Franciscan Rule and Franciscan spiritual directors, he came to lead a more balanced life.

During his life, the people of Urbino venerated John as a holy man and prophet.

John died on June 1, 1304, probably from effects of his severe lifestyle.

Pope Benedict XV proclaimed him Blessed on November 13, 1918.

Blessed John Pelingotto's feast day is June 2.

58

St. José Gabriel del Rosario Brochero, T.O.S.D.
March 16, 1840 – January 26, 1914

JOSÉ GABRIEL DEL ROSARIO BROCHERO was born on March 16, 1840 in Santa Rosa de Rio Primero, Córdoba, Argentina. He was the fourth of ten children. His family was very devout. In fact, his two sisters both became Religious Sisters.

When he was sixteen years old, José began studying to become a priest. During his early studies, he met Miguel Ángel Juárez-Celman, who would one day be the tenth President of Argentina.

In August of 1866, José became a member of the Third Order of St. Dominic, and was ordained a priest of the Archdiocese of Córdoba on November 4, 1866.

The year following his ordination, Fr. José found himself nursing the sick during a cholera epidemic. His heroic clinical nursing of infectious patients was only the first clue that this man was not afraid to serve people in any way he could.

One of his first assignments was as a prefect of studies at the seminary. On November 12, 1869, he received an advanced academic degree.

From even his early days as a priest, Fr. José showed a profound love for people and a strong desire to help them advance. Fortunately, he had the practicality of a good administrator and the energy and strength to carry out his plans. For example, to help people develop their spirituality, he founded a House of Exercise in 1877 and a school for girls in 1880.

What Fr. José was most famous for, however, was his many years as pastor of a vast, primitive rural area in Great Highlands region of Argentina. In his parish, which covered 1,675 square miles, Fr. José served 10,000 parishioners scattered all over the mountains and valleys.

Fr. José was a familiar figure among his flock, riding on horseback or by mule wearing his poncho and sombrero. The figure he cut led him to be known as "the gaucho" or "cowboy" priest.

Though his primary passion was to bring sacraments to the people, he strove as well to improve their physical lives. For example, Fr. José is credited with building postal stations, telegraph offices, and nearly 125 miles of roads, and helping officials plan for a railroad in the area.

Fr. José always had a special love for the sick and the poor, and one can almost imagine this religious cowboy figure arriving on his horse or donkey to give basic nursing care to people living in remote mountain and valley areas.

Somewhere along his pastoral journeys, Fr. José contracted Hansen's disease (leprosy). Some people thought Fr. José caught it from drinking *yerba mate* with lepers. (*Yerba mate* is a caffeinated drink that comes from a rainforest holly tree.) Others speculate he caught leprosy from nursing infected people.

Late in his life, Fr. José served at the Cathedral of Córdoba and later as pastor in Villa del Tránsito.

Fr. José, who eventually went blind and deaf, died on January 26, 1914. The cause of death was leprosy. His last words were, "Now I have everything ready for the journey."

Pope Francis canonized José Gabriel del Rosario Brochero on October 16, 2016. Pope Francis compared St. José Gabriel to the patron saint of priests, St. John Vianney, the Curé of Ars.

St. José Gabriel's feast day is January 26.

St. José Gabriel is a patron saint of Córdoba and its major seminary, clergy, and the Diocese of Cruz del Eje in Argentina.

59

Bl. José Tarrats Comaposada, S.J.
August 29, 1878 to September 28, 1936

José Tarrats Comaposada was born on August 29, 1878 in Barcelona, Spain.

When he grew up, Josep entered the Society of Jesus as a Jesuit Brother. José not only became the porter or doorkeeper of the house, but also nursed the sick of the community.

Brother José was martyred in the Spanish Civil War, killed on September 28, 1936 in his hometown of Barcelona.

Pope St. John Paul II beatified José on March 11, 2001.

Blessed José Tarrats Comaposada's feast day is September 28.

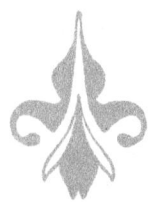

60

St. Joseph Benedict Cottolengo
May 3, 1786 – April 30, 1842

JOSEPH BENEDICT COTTOLENGO WAS BORN on May 3, 1786 in Bra, Cuneo Province, in the Piedmont area of the Kingdom of Sardinia – now Italy. He was the eldest of 12 children of a middle class family.

His mother, in particular, taught the children to have a special love for the sick and the poor. This obviously touched young Joseph, for when he was five years old, his family found him measuring his house. When asked why he was doing this, he replied that he wanted to find out how many sickbeds he could fit in the house so he could nurse the sick when he grew up.

Joseph was ordained a priest in Turin in 1811. After ordination, Fr. Joseph wanted nothing more than to be a parish priest in a simple country parish. His fellow priests, however, encouraged him to go on to further study. He followed their advice and received a degree in theology from the University of Turin.

After receiving his degree, he returned to his hometown to work for a few years as a priest. Then, in 1818, his bishop appointed him as canon of the Corpus Domini Basilica in Turin. He was to spend the rest of his life in Turin.

For eight or nine years, Fr. Joseph spent his time doing pastoral work in his parish in Turin. He also acquired the nickname "the good canon" for his love of the poor.

Fr. Joseph also became fascinated by the life of St. Vincent de Paul. He saw how much good Vincent had done in his life, and he began to think of devoting his life to the sick and the poor.

In 1827, Fr. Joseph had an experience that led him to finally make such a decision. A French family was passing through Turin on their way home. The family was very poor, and the mother was very sick. The general hospital in the town would not help her because she was pregnant, and the maternity hospital would not help her because she had tuberculosis. Therefore, the woman ended up in a room that the city provided for poor vagrants. There, she died while Fr. Joseph comforted her husband and children.

This incident led Fr. Joseph to devote the rest of his life to the sick and poor. He rented two rooms in a house across from the basilica to care for the sick, and later he rented more rooms. Though he had no grand plan for the future, Fr. Joseph trusted that Divine Providence would show him the way as he went along.

Unfortunately, the neighbors complained about the all the sick people coming to their neighborhood. Because cholera was being experienced in other parts of the Piedmont, city officials became afraid that the sick people coming to Fr. Joseph's place might bring it to their town. For these reasons, the city officials shut down Fr. Joseph's little hospital.

As a result, Fr. Joseph and his helpers went to a rundown place called Valdocco on the outskirts of Turin. In this district of shanties and taverns, they rented a small building. On April 27, 1832, the new building opened with just one patient – a man suffering from cancer. But in just a few months, Fr. Joseph needed to get another building to care for all the people who came to him. This was the beginning of what was to become known as the "Little House of Divine Providence." He put it under the patronage of St. Vincent de Paul. Fr. Joseph's motto was "The Love of Christ drives us forward."

Eventually, the houses began having specialized sections for the incurably ill, the infirm and aged, epileptics, the mentally ill, and sick and abandoned children.

The institution turned no one away. Fr. Joseph said, "All the poor are our patrons, but those who seem outwardly to be the most disgusting and repellent are our dearest patrons, indeed, are our jewels."

Fr. Joseph's little houses developed with shelters, orphanages, schools for the poor, workshops to teach trades, and, of course, hospitals for medical treatment and nursing care.

Because he could not do all the nursing himself, Fr. Joseph founded a confraternity of lay Brothers to help him, the Brothers of St. Vincent. He also founded a congregation called the Priests of the Holy Trinity to provide spiritual care for his charges. He also founded several congregations of Religious Sisters.

When nursing the sick, Fr. Joseph insisted that he and his fellow nurses care not only for the physical and mental health of their patients, but also for their spiritual well-being.

Fr. Joseph lived a very poor lifestyle to be "at one" with those he served.

To recognize Fr. Joseph for his amazing nursing and administrative works, King Charles Albert made him a Knight of the Order of Ss. Maurice and Lazarus.

Joseph died on April 30, 1842 in the main chapel in Valdocco.

Pope Pius XI canonized him in 1934.

St. Joseph Benedict Cottolengo's feast day is April 30.

61

St. Joseph Calasanz, Sch.P.
September 11, 1557 – August 25, 1648

Joseph Calasanz was born on September 11, 1557 in the Castle of Calasanz in Aragon (Spain), the youngest of eight children and the second of two boys. His father was a minor nobleman and mayor of the town.

In 1569, his parents sent Joseph to study at a school run by the Trinitarian friars. While there, he decided to become a priest.

Unfortunately, Joseph's parents opposed his wishes to be a priest, so Joseph continued his regular, secular studies.

He studied philosophy and law at the University of Lleida where he earned a Doctor of Laws degree, and then he studied theology at the University of Valencia and at Complutense University.

When Joseph's mother and his only brother died, Joseph's father wanted him to get married and have sons to carry on the family name. But in 1582, John became sick and almost died.

When Joseph recovered, his father felt relieved but guilty at having quashed Joseph's dreams. Therefore, Joseph's father gave his blessing for Joseph to pursue his dream of becoming a priest.

Joseph was ordained a priest on December 17, 1583. He served in various ministries in the Diocese of Albarracín as a procurator, theologian, and confessor. When his bishop was transferred to the Diocese of Lleida, Joseph followed him there.

After his bishop died, Joseph found himself as vicar general for the Bishop of Urgell. In 1592, at the age of 35, Joseph moved to Rome and worked as a theologian and spiritual director. In Rome, he fell in love with the poor, especially neglected and homeless boys who roamed the streets of the city.

Also in 1592, the plague entered Rome, and Joseph worked with his good friend, St. Camillus de Lellis (another Saintly Man of Nursing in this book), nursing the sick of the city.

Although Joseph did a fine job nursing the sick, nursing was not his lifelong passion as it was for Camillus. Therefore, while Camillus started a religious congregation to care for the sick, Joseph started a religious group devoted to the education of poor children.

Pope Clement VIII and Pope Paul V both heard of Fr. Joseph's work and helped him financially. Soon, Fr. Joseph found himself serving over a thousand poor children. In 1612 he moved his school, as he needed more room to expand and serve the ever-growing population of student who found their way to him.

Fr. Joseph is credited with founding the first free public school in Rome, and soon his Pious Schools, as they were known, spread all over Europe.

His religious community was known as the Congregation of Pious Schools. The Order's name was later changed to the Clerks Regular of the Christian Schools, in 1669. Members are commonly known as the Piarists or Scopoli.

While much of the teaching of the day was in Latin, Fr. Joseph insisted in also using the vernacular to teach. He also firmly believed in teaching with love instead of fear.

Because Fr. Joseph had a close friendship with Galileo, and because Galileo and his ideas were out of favor in his day, many people tried to condemn Joseph. He stuck by his friend, however, and ordered his fellow priests to treat Galileo with respect.

Unfortunately, Fr. Joseph's life became filled with deep sorrow because other Piarist priests' false accusations against him. In spite of every effort to ruin his reputation, Fr. Joseph remained faithful to his Lord and Church.

Fr. Joseph Calasanz died on August 25, 1648 in Rome at the age of 90.

Pope Clement XIII canonized him on July 16, 1767.

St. Joseph Calasanz is a patron saint of Catholic Schools. The feast day of St. Joseph Calasanz is August 25.

62

Bro. Joseph Dutton
April 27, 1843 – March 26, 1931

IRA DUTTON WAS BORN INTO a Protestant household on April 27, 1843 in Stowe, Vermont. When he was 18 years old, Ira was living in Wisconsin. There, he taught Sunday school and worked in a bookstore. Ira also liked to write about his life in journals.

When the Civil War broke out, Ira wrote about his excitement. In September of 1861, he enlisted in the Thirteenth Wisconsin Infantry Regiment fighting for the Union. Even though his regiment did not have many battle experiences, he rose to the rank of Captain.

Ira was discharged in 1866, because after the Civil War had ended, there was no need for so many people of his military rank.

When he got out of the army, Ira got married to a woman notorious for her promiscuity. His friends warned him against the marriage, but he wouldn't listen to them. In a short time, Ira discovered that his friends had been right. His wife cheated on him and was addicted to shopping. Not only did she run away with another man, she spent all of Ira's money. Ira kept hoping that one day she would return to him, but she never did. So he finally divorced her in 1881.

During the next two decades, Ira had many jobs. He worked in cemeteries, oversaw a distillery in Alabama, and worked on railroads in Memphis. In 1875, he joined the War Department settling claims that were brought against the government.

Though he was a good worker, Ira was what today we would call a "functioning alcoholic." Every night and weekend, he would drink alcohol to excess. In 1876, however, he had become so ashamed of his double life that he vowed never to drink again. This pledge he kept for the rest of his life. At his death, he could claim 55 years of continuous sobriety.

In 1883, on his fortieth birthday, Ira became a Catholic Christian and changed his name from "Ira" to "Joseph" in honor of his favorite saint. He then retired from government and set out to begin a new life. He wanted this new life to be one of penance for what he called his "wild years" and "sinful capers."

The first thing he did in his new life was to live at the Trappist monastery of Our Lady of Gethsemani, Kentucky for 20 months. But after this experience he concluded that to serve God more fully, he should live an active, apostolic life instead of a contemplative one. It was at this time that Joseph heard about the famous Father Damien, who was working with lepers on the island of Molokai in the Hawaiian Islands. He determined to give his life to help Fr. Damien.

In 1886, three years before Fr. Damien died, Joseph arrived, filled with the zeal that all missionaries feel when they begin their service. This intense missionary fire never left him.

Joseph soon found his way into the hearts of the people of Molokai. And though he never took vows as a religious Brother, people began calling him "Brother Joseph." They soon began relying on him for many things. Joseph was a jack-of-all-trades. In other words, he did what needed to be done. If Fr. Damien needed an administrator, Brother Joseph would be an administrator. Sometimes he would be a carpenter. Other times, he would nurse the sick and assist professional nurses in their duties. Other times he would be a repairman or a basketball coach or simply a consoler of the sick and the dying.

Just before he died, Fr. Damien – who is now known as Saint Damien (another Saintly Man of Nursing in this book) – told everyone that he could die in peace knowing that Brother Joseph was on hand to take his place.

Brother Joseph did continue Fr. Damien's work, always known for being a jovial and peaceful person. When he was 83 years old, Joseph wrote in his journal how his natural inclination was to be jolly. He reported that he was always ready to laugh, that a laugh was always just waiting to break out.

When people would ask him if he would like to take a vacation, he dismissed the idea. To him, nothing could be as happy or fulfilling as working on Molokai. For him, a vacation would feel more like a form of slavery.

Brother Joseph served the people of Molokai faithfully and joyfully for 45 years. Before his death, he wrote, "It has been a happy place – a happy life." Brother Joseph died on March 26, 1931.

Today, the Diocese of Honolulu is advancing Brother Joseph Dutton's cause for the journey to sainthood.

63

St. Joseph Freinademetz, S.V.D.
April 15, 1852 – January 28, 1908

JOSEPH FREINADEMETZ WAS BORN IN Oies, a tiny hamlet in the Dolomite Alps of northern Italy, on April 15, 1852 and was baptized the same day.

When he was a young man, Joseph decided to become a priest. While studying in the diocesan seminary, he began dreaming of one day becoming a foreign missionary.

Joseph was ordained a priest on July 25, 1873 and assigned to the parish of St. Martin, near his hometown. His parishioners loved him immediately.

Joseph learned, as others have learned through the ages, that once God puts the "missionary spirit" in a person, it never really leaves. Therefore, after two years of priesthood, Fr. Joseph contacted Fr. Arnold Janssen, founder of the Society of the Divine Word, an Order that focuses on missionary work.

Fr. Joseph entered the Order in the Netherlands in August 1878 to do his novitiate year.

One year later, on March 2, 1879, Joseph received his missionary cross and departed for China with Fr. John Baptist Anzer, another Divine Word Missionary.

Five weeks later, the two arrived in Hong Kong where they lived and studied Chinese culture and language for two years.

In 1881, Father Joseph and Fr. John Baptist left for their new mission in South Shantung province, a province with 12 million people. Of those 12 million, only 158 were Christian.

Father Joseph threw himself into missionary work with the zeal that all new missionaries have. He realized very early on how critical it was to train laypeople as catechists to teach the faith. Therefore, he put much energy into training catechists, even writing a manual in Chinese for them. He and Fr. Joseph spent much time working for the spiritual formation and ongoing education of the Chinese priests and other missionaries.

Eventually, Fr. John Baptist Anzer became a bishop.

Fr. Joseph's years in China were incredibly rewarding for him, and he absolutely loved the Chinese people. In fact, he once said that he would spend the rest of his life trying to be "a Chinese among the Chinese." Sociologists call this "going native," a phenomenon seen not only in missionaries, but also frequently seen in anthropologists and sociologists who do field research.

Though he was very fulfilled in his missionary work, these were hard years for Fr. Joseph. For example, he had to cope with assaults by bandits, long and arduous journeys, and the difficulties associated with forming new communities. In addition to all of those challenges, Fr. Joseph had to cope with continually starting over: whenever he would get a new Christian community going, the bishop would tell to him to leave everything and start anew somewhere else.

In 1898, Joseph became sick with laryngitis and early tuberculosis, in part caused from his heavy workload and hardships. Therefore, at the insistence of the bishop and fellow priests, he was sent to Japan for a well-deserved rest.

After his rest, he returned to China. Although he was not fully cured, Fr. Joseph threw himself into his work once again.

In 1907, the bishop had to leave the area on a journey, and he put Fr. Joseph in charge of the diocese until he returned. So Fr. Joseph not only had all of his regular missionary duties, he was now responsible for the daily administrative work of the diocese.

To add to those challenges, a typhoid epidemic then came to the diocese. Soon Fr. Joseph began nursing the sick as best he could, serving as a traveling nurse to the far-flung areas of the diocese. Not only did he do biophysical and what we would today call psychosocial nursing, he made sure the patients received the sacraments. As a result of his nursing the sick, Fr. Joseph himself became infected.

Fr. Joseph returned to Taikia, the seat of the diocese, and died on January 28, 1908. He was buried at the twelfth station on the Way of the Cross, and soon his grave became a site for Christian pilgrims.

Pope St. John Paul II canonized Fr. Joseph on October 5, 2003.

St. Joseph Freinademetz' feast day is January 28.

64

Bl. Joseph Gerard, O.M.I.
March 12, 1831 – May 29, 1914

JOSEPH GERARD WAS BORN ON March 12, 1831 near Nancy, France.

He spent his childhood on the family farm. With the help of a parish priest, Joseph was able to enter the seminary to study for the priesthood. While still a seminarian, Joseph learned of a newly established missionary society – the Missionary Oblates of Mary Immaculate (OMI). Awed by inspirational missionary tales of adventure, Joseph decided to join their congregation.

When he was 22 years old, the founder of the Oblates, Blessed Eugene de Mazenod, ordained Joseph a deacon and gave him his first assignment as a missionary - a mission in Natal in South Africa.

In May of 1853, Deacon Joseph set out for Africa, never to see France again.

On February 19, 1854, Joseph was ordained a priest in South Africa. His special ministry was to work with the Zulu people, but he also worked with the local European population.

Fr. Joseph spent very hard years working in the area, journeying through the rough countryside, learning new languages, dealing with intense heat and cold, and often sleeping outdoors. He became very discouraged, for despite his love and care and diligence, his work didn't seem to bear much fruit. Only later would he learn that the seeds he planted in the hearts of the Zulu people would flourish and bloom.

In 1862, he went to Basutoland (now Lesotho) to work with the Basotho people, hoping to have more success than he had with the Zulu people. He labored as a missionary in Lesotho for the next 52 years.

It took Fr. Joseph two years of hard work before he made his first convert among the Basotho people. However, within five years, a new congregation of Sisters began, and he established a successful mission station in Roma, Basutoland. Today this area has many novitiates and seminaries, high schools, an Oblate university, religious houses, and a hospital. The people attribute all of these successes to the seeds planted by Fr. Joseph.

But of all the work Fr. Joseph did, his greatest love was caring for the sick. In fact, many reports say his nursing care – both biophysical and what we would now call psychosocial – was heroic. Long distances, treacherous mountain trails, and terrible weather could not stop him from making sick calls either on foot on by horse.

Fr. Joseph spent his last years at the mission in Roma. He continued caring for the sick no matter where they were, even when his arthritis bent him over almost in half, his sight was nearly gone, and he had to be lifted up onto his faithful horse Artaban.

Up to a month before his death, at the age of 83, Fr. Joseph could be seen making nursing rounds to care for those in need.

Fr. Joseph died on May 29, 1914.

Pope St. John Paul II beatified him on September 15, 1988.

Blessed Joseph Gerard's feast day is May 29.

65

St. Joseph Oriol
November 23, 1650 – March 23, 1702

JOSEPH ORIOL WAS BORN ON November 23, 1650 in Barcelona to a poor silk-weaver and his wife. His father died when Joseph was just six months old. His mother married again, and her new husband, a cobbler, loved his stepson very much.

Joseph's parents sent him to their parish church, St. Mary's by the Sea, for his basic education. In the parish, Joseph served as a catechist, altar server, and choir member. He eventually became the parish's sacristan, and he loved spending time with the Blessed Sacrament.

When Joseph was 12 or 13, his stepfather died. To ease the burden on his widowed mother, Joseph went to live with Caterina Brugera, the woman who had nursed him as a baby. He lived with Caterina for the next 13 years.

During his time in Caterina's home, Joseph spent his time studying at the University of Barcelona, thanks to the generosity of an anonymous donor. When he was 23, Joseph received a doctorate in theology and then went on to study Hebrew and moral theology.

In 1676, Joseph was ordained to the priesthood. Because his mother was always in need of financial support, Fr. Joseph took a job as a tutor in the home of a very wealthy family. This home was a far cry from his poor beginnings, but he tried to adjust to this lavish place. However, in 1677, an amazing conversion experience happened to Fr. Joseph. As he was dining one day, and about to serve himself from an abundant bowl of food, he felt an invisible hand hold his hand back from taking his portion. This happened not just once, but three times. Fr. Joseph interpreted this as a divine sign that the "high life" he was living was not his calling.

As a result of this experience, Fr. Joseph decided to undertake a lifelong fast, taking only bran bread and water. On special feast days, he would add a few herbs to his bread, and on Christmas and Easter, he would add one sardine to his diet. He stayed with the wealthy family until his mother's death in 1686.

Joseph's diet was not the only unusual thing about his spirituality. After leaving the luxurious home where he had been a tutor, he rented an attic room that had only a table, chair, crucifix, and a few books. There, he would pray and flagellate himself nightly. He had no fire to keep him warm in the winters, and he wore the same raggedy clothes in all seasons. He tried to detach himself from all material comforts, giving himself totally to God.

Initially people made fun of him on the streets. However, as they got to know this holy man, they began to love him. Children, for example, would run up to kiss his hands, and he would lead them to church for a catechism lesson. Women were said to treat him more as an angel than a man.

Fr. Joseph had a special influence over soldiers and prisoners, because he was always very kind to them. One of Fr. Joseph's greatest gifts was his respectful listening to anyone who came to him. Even street vendors and tradesmen would rise as a sign of respect as he passed along the streets.

In spite of his incredible asceticism and severe lifestyle, Joseph was never morose. On the contrary, he was known as an incredibly joyful man, radiating Christ to all he encountered.

Fr. Joseph, who is said to have the gift of reading souls, was a popular confessor, and he gave much of his time to this sacrament.

Despite Fr. Joseph's wonderful work in Barcelona, he became convinced of a need to become a martyr. Therefore, he decided to go to Rome to ask to be sent to the foreign missions. He was begged by all not to leave, but left anyway. However, when he got to Marseilles, he had a vision of the Virgin Mary telling him to return to Barcelona. He did so, and at that time decided to devote the rest of his life to nursing the sick.

Soon his fame spread far and wide. People would flock to his church where he would dip his fingers into holy water and make the sign of the cross or lay his hands on them. Many people reported miraculous cures as a result of Fr. Joseph's interventions. The only people who were not happy with Fr. Joseph were the pharmacists who were losing business because of his cures.

In 1702, sensing the end was near, Fr. Joseph moved out of his rented attic and moved to a room with a friend. As death approached, he had the Sacrament of the Sick, gazed at the crucifix, and died. This was on March 23, 1702.

Immense crowds flocked to Fr. Joseph's funeral bier. In fact, so many people came to his funeral that the officials had to close the church doors to allow the funeral Mass to take place.

Pope St. Pius X canonized Joseph Oriol on May 20, 1909.

St. Joseph Oriol's feast day is March 23.

66

Bl. Juan Agustín Codera-Marqués, S.D.B.
May 25, 1883 – September 25, 1936

JUAN AGUSTÍN CODERA-MARQUÉS WAS BORN on May 25, 1883 in Barbastro, Huesca, Spain.

In his thirties he joined the Salesians of St. Don Bosco. Juan Agustín took his vows on July 24, 1919 in Carabanchel Alto in Madrid.

Juan devoted himself to nursing. Unfortunately, his nursing career was interrupted many times by being arrested during the Spanish Civil War. One day he was apprehended on his way to visit the sick. The Nationalist authorities shot him on September 25, 1936 in Madrid, Spain.

On June 26, 2006, Pope Benedict XVI declared Juan Agustín to be a martyr, and on October 28, 2007, the same Pope beatified him.

Blessed Juan Agustín Codera-Marqués' feast day is September 25.

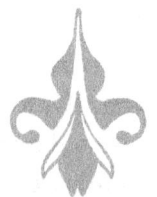

67

Bl. Juan Bautista Egozcuezábal-Aldaz, O.H.
March 13, 1882 – July 29, 1936

JUAN BAUTISTA EGOZCUEZÁBAL-ALDAZ WAS BORN on March 13, 1882 in Nuin, Navarra, Spain.

When he was 29 years old, he joined the Carmelites on January 31, 1911. He transferred to the Hospitallers of St. John of God when he was 30.

Juan Bautista worked for a time as a psychiatric-mental health nurse, and later as a nurse for handicapped children.

One day, as he was leaving the children's hospital, Spanish Nationalist authorities captured him and ordered him to denounce Christianity. When he refused, the officials fatally shot him on July 29, 1936 in Barcelona and threw his body in a field in Espulgues de Llobregat.

Pope St. John Paul II beatified Juan on October 25, 1992.

Blessed Juan's feast day is July 29. He is also celebrated as part of the Martyred Hospitallers of Spain's feast day, July 30.

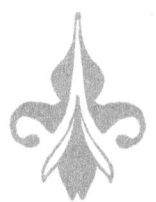

68

St. Juan Macías, O.P.
March 2, 1585 – September 16, 1645

JUAN DE ARCAS Y SÁNCHEZ was born was born on March 2, 1585 in Ribera del Fresno, Extremadura, Spain. Juan's parents were poor farmers who died when Juan and his sister Agnes were very young. Because their uncle raised them, both children took their uncle's family name as their own – Macías. Juan's uncle trained him to be a shepherd.

When he was 16 years old, Juan met a Dominican friar in a neighboring village, and began considering becoming a friar himself one day.

At the age of 25, Juan went to work for a rich businessman who offered him the opportunity to go to South America. Juan jumped at the chance and in 1610, he left Spain and landed at Cartagena, Colombia and eventually made his way to Peru. There, he worked for a time on a cattle ranch and did other jobs, and he saved his money. He made his way to Lima, where he would spend the rest of his life.

In January of 1622, Juan entered the Dominican friary of St. Mary Magdalene in Lima as a lay brother. He gave all of his savings to the Order. One year later, in January of 1623, he took his vows. Interestingly, he was a contemporary of another lay Dominican brother in a different monastery – Martin de Porres – who is also listed as a Saintly Man of Nursing in this book.

In his own priory, Juan served as the doorkeeper until his death. Like Martin, Juan showed the world how important the role of porter or doorkeeper could be. Though he would have loved to live more as a hermit, he accepted his role of greeting the public with grace, energy, and joy.

Soon the doors of the priory became a gathering place for the sick, poor, and needy of the city. Brother Juan not only nursed the sick who came to him, he made sure all who came to him in need would get food and clothes if they needed them.

Brother Juan's nursing care was not limited to the poor, and it was not limited to biophysical nursing. He also did what would now be called psychosocial nursing for the rich and famous who would come to him for counseling.

To help him in his work, Brother Juan trained a donkey to "make rounds" in the city for him. Equipped with large panniers, the donkey would go from store to store, house to house. People became familiar with the donkey and would put food, wine, clothes, money, or whatever they had to offer, in the panniers. If people didn't show up at the door of their house or business, the donkey would make a lot of noise to get their intention. After collecting what it could, the donkey would return home to Brother Juan to deliver its collection.

In Juan's day, many people attributed healing miracles to him – not only from his nursing care, but also from his prayers. After his death, miracles continued to be attributed to him. It is little wonder that Juan became known as "the father of the poor" in Peru.

Brother Juan died on September 16, 1645, and all of Lima mourned his loss.

Pope Paul VI canonized Juan Macías in 1975.

St. Juan Macías' feast day is September 16.

69

Bro. Juan de Mena, O.P.
Died 1554

Juan de Mena, not to be confused with a fifteenth-century Spanish poet of the same name, was a Dominican lay brother from Mexico. His brother, Marcos de Mena, was also a Dominican lay brother.

For reasons that are unclear, the two brothers, along with four other Dominican friars, were talked into leaving their Mexican province and going to Spain. Unfortunately, their ship was shipwrecked on Padre Island in what is now Texas.

Indians shot Brother Marcos with seven arrows, and he was left for dead. Fortunately, he recovered and thirty years later gave an account of the bloody day in 1554 when the shipwreck occurred.

Brother Juan was not so fortunate. After being shot in the back with an arrow, he tried to keep up with the other survivors, but he soon died from his wound.

Brother Juan, who was noted for his extraordinary compassion for the sick and his nursing skills, was known as "Mexico's nurse." He is given the honor of being the first nurse in the land that would one day be known as the United States of America.

70

St. Justin de Jacobis, C.M.
October 9, 1800 – July 31, 1860

JUSTIN DE JACOBIS WAS BORN on October 9, 1800 in San Fele in southern Italy, but his family later moved to Naples.

When Justin was 18 years old, a Carmelite priest encouraged him to enter the Congregation of the Missions, otherwise known as the Vincentians. Justin followed this priest's suggestion, and in 1924 he was ordained a priest. Following his ordination, Fr. Justin became well known as a preacher and confessor, and he showed great administrative ability.

In 1836, Fr. Justin returned to Naples just when the city was hit by a devastating cholera epidemic. Fr. Justin immediately began nursing the sick of the city and showed outstanding compassion and charity in this work. He especially loved to care for the poor who had been infected.

Because Fr. Justin had expressed a desire to become a foreign missionary, his superiors chose him to lead a group of missionaries to Ethiopia. On May 24, 1839, Fr. Justin began his journey and arrived in Adowa on October 13. There, he met the founder of the mission and did all he could to learn about the country.

Justin learned, for example, that the majority Catholic Christians were of the Coptic Rite, and that the Coptic Rite priests were often hostile toward the Latin Rite priests. He also learned that Latin Rite priests had been banned in that country since 1632, and that this Vincentian mission was the first to be established since then. It was in this context of drama and hostility that Fr. Justin began his missionary endeavors.

Fr. Justin, in contrast to many of the other Latin Rite priests, believed that whenever possible, the liturgy should be celebrated in the Coptic Rite. He continually argued for an indigenous clergy, preferring poorly instructed Ethiopian priests to highly educated European ones. This emphasis on a native clergy is a mark of the genuine missionary.

Over his protests, Justin was secretly consecrated a bishop in 1848. Because the government was hostile to the work of the Church, especially toward the Latin Rite Catholics, Bishop Justin tried to be as inconspicuous as possible. At one time in 1854, he was arrested and suffered for the Faith, but was released when some of the clergy ransomed him from captivity.

In 1858, Bishop Justin found himself once again nursing the sick in a cholera epidemic that came to Gondar where he was living.

On July 31, 1860, Justin died in the desert from a fever.

Although Bishop Justin was noted for his administrative skills and other missionary qualities, everyone who knew him most strongly remembered his great humility.

Pope Paul VI canonized Justin de Jacobis on October 26, 1975.

St. Justin de Jacobis' feast day is July 31.

71
Bl. Liberatus Weiss, O.F.M.
January 4, 1675 – March 3, 1716

JOHANNES LAURENTIUS WEISS WAS BORN on January 4, 1675 in Konnersreuth, Bavaria, second of six children.

Although he went to Cistercian schools, Johannes became attracted to the Franciscans who frequently came to his town to preach.

On October 13, 1693, Johannes was received into the Franciscan Order in Ganz and received the name Liberatus.

He was ordained to the priesthood in 1698 and served in parish ministry in Langenlois until 1703 when he became a city preacher in Ganz. While serving in Ganz, his superior asked him to become a missionary to Ethiopia. The ruler of Ethiopia, Jasu, had requested that a team be sent there, and Liberatus was made the superior of this expeditionary missionary group.

Fr. Liberatus was accepted by the Society for the Propagation of the Faith as a missionary to Ethiopia. He took with him seven priests and three lay brothers. After a treacherous journey, they reached present-day Khartoum, where the local ruler refused to welcome them. In fact, he robbed the group of all of their possessions, and all but two of the missionaries died – Fr. Liberatus and Fr. Michael Pius (who is also a Saintly Man of Nursing in this book).

Dejected, the two men fled to Egypt for safety. However, in the fall of 1711, Father Liberatus took Fr. Michael Pius with him back to Ethiopia, along with Fr. Samuel Marzorati (another Saintly Man of Nursing in this book).

They arrived in Massawa on April 18, 1712, and then traveled to the capital of Gonder where they arrived in July 1712.

Though the ruler there welcomed them, he would not allow them to publicly preach because of his precarious hold on political power. Therefore, Fathers Liberatus, Michael, and Samuel built a hospital where they nursed the sick while learning the language and cultural customs of the people. They continued their nursing for three years.

Unfortunately for everyone, the three men were never to begin the preaching ministry for which they were sent to Ethiopia. They refused to give their assent to heretical teaching, and were sentenced to death. Liberatus and his companions spent the night before their execution singing sacred hymns. They were stoned to death on March 3, 1716 at a place called Abbo, a place of execution.

Pope St. John Paul II beatified Fr. Liberatus and his companions on November 20, 1988.

Blessed Liberatus and companions' feast day is March 3.

72

Bl. Luchesio Modestini, O.F.S.
c. 1180 – April 28, 1260

LUCHESIO MODESTINI WAS BORN SOMETIME between 1180 and 1182 in Gaggiano near Milan, Lombardy.

As a young man, he became a merchant. Unfortunately, he became obsessed with making money. In fact, he developed a reputation in his town as an avaricious man. His wife, Buonadonna, also highly coveted material possessions.

Sometime in his thirties, Luchesio had a spiritual conversion, and his wife followed suit. Luchesio came to realize how foolish his materialistic nature had been.

Luchesio put on a gray tunic – which was a symbol of a penitent in those days – and began to devote himself to an ascetic lifestyle. For example, it was not uncommon for him to fast on bread and water and sleep on the hard floor.

Luchesio began to put his faith into action by nursing the sick and visiting those in prison. He also gave away all his possessions and land except for a small a small piece of land necessary to cultivate crops to feed for his wife and himself.

Though Luchesio and Buonadonna thought about leaving each other and joining religious orders, they decided to live as a married couple and grow in holiness in that vocation. Some writers believe that St. Francis of Assisi, who knew Luchesio before his conversion, may have encouraged them to stay together.

When Francis told the couple that he was planning on starting an Order for laypersons, they both asked to be received into it immediately. St. Francis granted their wish, and Luchesio and his wife became part of the Franciscan Order of Penance – today known as the Secular Franciscan Order. Some believe Luchesio and Buonadonna were the first tertiaries – or members of this Order – but that is not certain.

Luchesio often gave away all the food in their house to feed his patients he was nursing and the poor. But he never worried, for he figured that if Jesus could feed thousands, Jesus could put some more food in the pantry.

Not only did Luchesio nurse the sick in his home, he sometimes actually carried sick people to his home for nursing care.

During his life, Luchesio had frequent ecstasies and was noted for a gift of healing. One day, for example, Luchesio was carrying a sick and lame man to his home to be nursed. A young man saw this and mockingly asked, "What poor devil is that you are carrying on your back?" Luchesio calmly replied, "I am carrying my Lord Jesus Christ." At that, the young man's face became distorted, and he cried out fearfully and was struck dumb. He threw himself to his knees in front of Luchesio in contrition. Luchesio made the Sign of the Cross over the young man, and the young man was restored to speech.

When Luchesio became very ill with a fever, his wife begged him not to die before her. She argued that just as God had given them to each other as companions in life, God should permit them to die together.

God heard Buonadonna's prayers, and after receiving the sacraments, Luchesio and Buonadonna both died on April 28, 1260.

Pope Gregory X beatified Luchesio and Buonadonna in 1274.

Blessed Luchesio Modestini's feast day is April 28.

73

St. Louis Bertrán, O.P.
January 1, 1526 – October 9, 1581

LOUIS BERTRÁN WAS BORN ON January 1, 1526 in Valencia, Spain in a family of nine children.

In August of 1539, at the age of 18, Louis joined the Order of Preachers (Dominicans) at St. Dominic Convent in Valencia. According to biographers, Louis did not have much of a sense of humor, and his presentation of himself was rather stiff. However, when people got to know him, they discovered that Louis had a very sweet disposition, and they liked him very much.

Though Louis was not a very good student, he studied hard and was able to master his subjects.

The Archbishop of Valencia, St. Thomas of Villanova, ordained Louis a priest in 1547.

Fr. Louis immediately became master of novices in the Valencia house. He served in this position on and off for a total of 30 years.

When a plague broke out in Valencia in 1557, Fr. Louis devoted himself to nursing the sick and burying the dead. He even prepared bodies for burial, and indeed, dug graves and buried the people himself.

It was through his amazing nursing care that led people to identify Fr. Louis with great holiness.

One day, the great Carmelite saint, Teresa of Avila, approached him to ask for his advice. She had been planning to reform the Carmelite Order, and she wanted Louis' opinion. He encouraged her to go ahead with the project. In fact, he predicted that one day her new Order, which would become known as the Discalced (barefoot) Carmelites, would one day be one of the most famous Orders in the Church.

In 1562, Fr. Louis went to South America to help lead the people to Jesus. He began his work in Colombia, and soon became known as a miracle worker. He converted thousands of people by his preaching and his humble lifestyle.

From reports of Fr. Louis' life, it appears that part of his success was due to his having the gift of tongues. This manifested itself when Indian people of languages other than Spanish could still understand his preaching.

He also worked for a time in the Leeward, Virgin, and Windward Islands.

Though he was highly successful in making converts, Fr. Louis' missionary life was not problem-free. For example, the Carib tribe in the Leeward Islands tried once to poison him.

Fr. Louis returned to Spain after six years. He reported to the Spanish government what he had learned in the New World. He told of the cruelty and greed of many of the Spaniard settlers and how badly they treated the people of South America. No longer could Spanish government officials plead ignorance.

Fr. Louis spent the rest of his life training future missionaries. He always stressed to them that the only effective way to get ready for preaching was by humble and fervent prayer, and that words without works have no power to change people's lives.

Fr. Louis died in Valencia after a long illness on October 9, 1581.

Pope Clement X canonized him on April 12, 1671.

St. Louis Bertrán's feast day is October 9.

St. Louis Bertrán is a patron saint of Colombia, Dominican novices, and Caribbean vicariates.

74

St. Ludovico of Casoria, O.F.M.
March 11, 1814 – March 30, 1885

ARCHANGELO PALMENTIERI WAS BORN ON March 11, 1814 in Casoria, a town near Naples in what is now Italy.

As a youth, he was an apprentice for a cabinetmaker. However, in 1832 he gave up his career to enter the Franciscan Order of Friars Minor, taking the name Ludovico. Five years later, he was ordained a priest. His first assignment was to teach philosophy, chemistry, and mathematics to the younger members of his Order at St. Peter Priory in Naples.

In 1854, Fr. Ludovico experienced a mystical experience that he called a "cleansing." Following this event, he devoted his entire life to the sick and the poor. One of the first acts in his new life was to establish an infirmary called "La Palma," where he nursed the ill friars of his community.

Fr. Ludovico's love and passion for serving those in need, however, was much too expansive for one infirmary. Therefore, he used his remarkable energy and skills to embark on a life of amazing accomplishments. Rather than devoting himself solely to clinical nursing, he established many institutions.

Among his foundations was a dispensary for the poor, two schools for African children, an institute for children of nobility, an orphanage, an institution for the deaf and mute, and institutions for the blind, elderly, and travelers. These institutions were established in many cities, including Naples, Florence, and Assisi. He also fostered vocations to Africa and established an organization for the ransom and Christian formation of African children who had been sold as slaves.

Like other men who found themselves called to nurse the sick, Fr. Ludovico knew that he could make the most impact if he enlisted others to pursue his work. Therefore, he founded two religious communities. The first community was called the Gray Brothers (because of their gray habit). The men of this Order were former members of the Secular Franciscan Order. The second group he founded was the Gray Sisters of St. Elizabeth.

Through his institutions and religious communities, Fr. Ludovico expanded his nursing love to many thousands.

Around 1876, Fr. Ludovico contracted a serious and painful illness, from which he never completely recovered. On March 30, 1885, he died in the Marine Hospital in Posillipo, a residential district of Naples.

Within five months after Fr. Ludovico's death, his followers began preparing for his eventual canonization.

Pope Francis canonized Ludovico of Casoria on November 23, 2014.

St. Ludovico of Casoria's feast day is March 30. He is the patron saint of Casoria, Italy.

75

Bl. Luigi Maria Monti, C.F.I.C.
July 24, 1825 – October 1, 1900

LUIGI MARIA MONTI WAS BORN on July 24, 1825 in Bovisio Masciago, a city in the Diocese of Milan, Italy. He was the eighth of 11 children.

When Luigi was 12 years old, his father died. To help support the family, Luigi began making woodcrafts to sell in the market.

In the evenings, Luigi gathered together other devout craftsmen and farmers in his shop for prayer. Although the locals called his prayer group *The Company of Friars*, its official name was *The Company of the Sacred Heart of Jesus*.

The primary work of the group, in addition to prayer, was to evangelize lapsed Catholics and bring them back to the practice of their faith. Eventually the group expanded its mission to include working with the sick and the poor.

In 1846, Luigi took private vows of chastity and obedience and dedicated his life to God. Perhaps he made his vows in front of his spiritual director, Fr. Luigi Dossi.

During those years, there was much political turmoil in Italy. Some in the town spread the rumor that Luigi and his group were actually functionaries of the occupying Austrian forces. As a result, Luigi and his little group were arrested and put in jail in Milan. Fortunately, after six weeks government officials released Luigi and the rest of the group when it was acknowledged that they were indeed a religious group, not a political one.

When Fr. Dossi joined a new religious community called the Sons of Mary Immaculate, Luigi Monti followed him. Blessed Lodovico Pavoni had founded this community only five years earlier.

Luigi spent six years in Congregation of the Sons of Mary Immaculate as a layman. During this time, he studied nursing theory and gained clinical nursing experience in Brescia during the cholera epidemic of 1855. He also volunteered to be isolated with patients in an asylum for the sick.

Eventually Luigi, along with his spiritual director Fr. Luigi Dossi, left the congregation to establish a new congregation dedicated to caring for the sick. Luigi envisioned this group of men to have both clerical and lay members, all equal in rights and responsibilities. In 1877, with the help of Pope Blessed Pius IX, Luigi established *The Congregation of the Sons of the Immaculate Conception*. Pius IX approved the Order. Luigi, though he would remain a layman for his entire life, served as the Order's leader for as long he lived. The members often called him "Father Luigi" even though he was not a priest.

The men of this new Order were amazing and heroic nurses. They were never afraid to minister during epidemics to serve the sick, often serving in places where other nurses were afraid to go.

Luigi founded houses of his Order throughout the region. His men nursed the sick in local hospitals, also using their houses as centers from which they would travel as visiting nurses to remote villages and farms.

The Sons of the Immaculate Conception were very focused on nursing the sick. However, in 1882, Luigi had an experience that led him to expand the mission of the Order to include working with orphaned children. One day, a Carthusian monk showed up with his four nephews in tow. The boys had lost both parents and had no one to care for them. Their story touched Luigi's heart immensely, and he determined not only to build an orphanage, but to make the care of orphans one his Order's missions.

Luigi Monti died on October 1, 1900 at the age of 75, totally exhausted from his active life.

Pope St. John Paul II beatified Luigi Maria Monti on November 9, 2003. Blessed Luigi Maria Monti's feast day is October 1.

76

Bl. Luke Belludi, O.F.M.
1200 – c. 1285

LUKE BELLUDI WAS BORN SOMETIME in 1200 to a wealthy family in Padua, in what is now Italy.

One day, when St. Anthony of Padua was preaching in the city, Luke came up to him and asked if he could join the newly formed Friars Minor (which came to be called Franciscans). Anthony was quite impressed with this 20-year-old man, so he introduced Luke to St. Francis of Assisi himself. Francis liked young Luke and accepted him into his Order.

Francis assigned young Luke to accompany St. Anthony in his travels. Little did Anthony know that Luke was to become the most important person in his life.

When Anthony journeyed from one place to another, Luke accompanied him. When it came time for Anthony to die, Luke served him as a private duty nurse.

On the death of Anthony, Luke took his place in the Order.

He was given the task of being the guardian of the Franciscans in Padua. Unfortunately for Luke, calamity was just around the corner.

In 1239, the City of Padua fell into the hands of evil men bent on destruction. Soon, noblemen were killed, the mayor and council were banished, and the University of Padua was closed. The construction of a basilica in honor of St. Anthony of Padua was stopped, and Luke himself was banished from the city. That, however, did not stop him, for in the dark of night, he would sneak back into the city and go to the unfinished basilica with the new guardian of the Franciscans.

One night, while Luke and his companion were in the unfinished basilica, they heard a voice assuring them that the city would soon be delivered from the evil tyrants, which indeed happened.

When the city was back to normal, and Luke had become the Provincial Minister of the Franciscans, he finished the basilica dedicated to his mentor, friend, and patient, St. Anthony.

Luke went on to establish many Franciscan institutions, and like his mentor, St. Anthony, he was considered to be a miracle worker.

Luke died around 1285. He was buried in the basilica, side by side with St. Anthony.

Blessed Luke Belludi's feast day is February 24.

77

St. Martin de Porres, O.P.
December 9, 1579 – November 3, 1639

JUAN MARTIN DE PORRES-VELÁSQUEZ WAS born in Lima, Peru on December 9, 1579. His father was a Spanish nobleman, and his mother was a freed slave from Panama. Because the father was disappointed that his son had dark skin like his mother, he insisted that official papers have "son of an unknown father" listed. Two years later, the couple produced a second child, Juana.

The family lived in poverty. To make ends meet, Martin's mother tried to keep the family together by taking in laundry. Martin and Juana's father took them to Ecuador with him to gain some education, but when Martin was around 12 years old, the father sent the children back to their mother. At that time, Martin was apprenticed to a surgeon-barber in Lima and learned how to care for wounds and fractures and how to prescribe medicines. He also gained some pharmaceutical knowledge from his mother, who was a practitioner of herbal medicine.

When he was 16, Martin entered the Convent of the Holy Rosary as a *donado*, a member of the Third Order of St. Dominic who could live in the convent and do menial work. Martin's father, who was now the Governor of Panama, was outraged, for he saw the role of *donado* as too menial. Though he insisted Martin be accepted as a full member of the Order, that request was denied. In the first place, there was a law forbidding "Indians, blacks, and their descendants" from joining religious Orders, but additionally, Martin himself felt unworthy to be a member. In 1603, however, the superiors decided to ignore the law and profess Martin as a lay brother.

As a Brother, Martin did many jobs in the convent. However, he was most noted for his role as infirmarian of the community, a role he held until his death. In this role, he nursed the sick of the Dominican community with great compassion, sensitivity, and skill.

Brother Martin nursed not only the sick of his Order, but also people of the larger community, from slaves to noblemen. One time, for example, he gave up his own bed to treat an old beggar covered with ulcers. When one of the other Brothers reproved him, Martin said, "Compassion, my dear Brother, is preferable to cleanliness."

Brother Martin also took the lead in caring for friars who became ill in an epidemic. To protect the professed members from the novices who were infected with the disease, doors were locked. Martin, however, was seen miraculously passing through locked doors in order to nurse the novices, as though he were a ghost.

Martin was also famous for feeding the hungry that came to the convent. In fact, in normal times, he fed 160 poor people every day at the convent. In addition, he also founded an orphanage for abandoned children in the City of Lima.

Despite his untiring work in the convent and community, Martin did not confine his nursing skills to human beings. He also had great love for animals, and he cared for dogs and cats that were in need, establishing an animal hospital at his sister's house.

Brother Martin was also a friend of two other extraordinary people who lived in Lima at the time – St. Rose of Lima and St. Juan Macías. Juan Macías, who is also a Saintly Man of Nursing in this book, was a Brother in a different Dominican house of the city.

Though Brother Martin was noted for his remarkable nursing spirit and practice, he was also known for supernatural gifts. For example, often when he was in deep prayer, others saw his body floating above the floor and a great light flooding his room. He was also blessed with the gift of bilocation, the ability to be in more than one place at a time. Though he only lived in Peru and Ecuador, people reported seeing him in Africa, China, Mexico, Algeria, and Japan.

Brother Martin de Porres died on November 3, 1639. The whole city of Lima mourned his death.

Pope St. John XXIII canonized Martin de Porres on May 6, 1962.

St. Martin de Porres' feast day is November 3.

St. Martin de Porres is a patron saint of barbers, nurses, people of mixed races, public health workers, innkeepers, African-Americans, hairdressers, social justice, television, and others.

78

Bl. Michael Pius Fasoli, O.F.M.
May 3, 1676 – March 3, 1716

MICHAEL PIUS FASOLI WAS BORN on May 3, 1676 in Zerbo, Lombardy.

When he was a young adult, he became a Franciscan and agreed to join Fr. Liberatus Weiss (another Saintly Man of Nursing in this book) to be a missionary in Ethiopia.

In September of 1704, a missionary group, headed by Fr. Liberatus, set out for Ethiopia, full of dreams for accomplishing great things for Christ. This group comprised eight priests and three lay brothers.

Tragically, when the group reached present-day Khartoum, the ruler of the area robbed them of all their belongings. Of the original group of eleven men, all died of starvation except for Fathers Liberatus and Michael Pius.

After fleeing to Egypt, Fathers Liberatus and Michael Pius took on a third priest, Fr. Samuel Marzorati (another Saintly Man of Nursing in this book), and headed back to Ethiopia.

In Ethiopia, the local ruler gave them a lukewarm welcome. While he allowed them to stay, he did not allow them to preach in public. Therefore, the men started a little hospital where they nursed the sick of the area. In addition to their nursing duties, they also studied the cultural customs and language of the people so that one day, they might become excellent missionaries.

Unfortunately, that day never came, for the government sentenced them to be stoned to death before ever being able to preach the good news of Jesus Christ.

The night before their martyrdom, they spent the whole night singing sacred hymns. When day came, they were taken to the place of execution – Abbo – on March 3, 1716. There they were stoned to death.

Pope St. John Paul II beatified Michael Pius Fasoli and his companions on November 20, 1988.

St. Michael Pius Fasoli and companions' feast day is March 3.

79

St. Michael Kozaki, O.F.S.
c. 1551 – February 5, 1597

MICHAEL KOZAKI WAS A LAYMAN born in Japan around 1551.

Michael was a bow maker and carpenter. When Franciscan missionaries arrived in the area in which he lived, Michael was already a Catholic Christian. He became a Secular Franciscan and worked with the Franciscans as a catechist. He also worked as a nurse in the hospital they established.

His carpentry skills were useful to build convents and churches in Kyoto and Osaka.

On February 5, 1597, Michael – along with 25 other Catholic Christians - was crucified at Tateyama (Hill of Wheat) in Nagasaki, Japan. Michael's 14-year old son, St. Thomas Kozaki, was one of the 26 people martyred that day. Michael was 46 years old.

Pope Urban VIII canonized Michael and Thomas along with 24 other martyrs, all known as the Martyrs of Nagasaki, on June 8, 1862.

The feast day of the Martyrs of Nagasaki is February 6.

80

Bl. Michael Rua, S.D.B.
June 9, 1837 – April 6, 1910

MICHAEL RUA WAS BORN IN a poverty-stricken neighborhood of Turin, Piedmont, on June 9, 1837. He was the youngest of nine children. His father, who was a supervisor in a weapons factory, died when Michael was just eight years old.

As a child, Michael attended a school run by the Brothers of Christian Schools. It was in that school's poor neighborhood that young Michael met an amazing priest named John Bosco, a man who is also a Saintly Man of Nursing in this book. Fr. Bosco had a passion to help poor boys get a good schooling and a good start on life. Eventually, Fr. Bosco founded a religious community, which he named after one of his heroes, St. Francis de Sales. Its members were called Salesians.

In 1845, Fr. Bosco enlisted Michael to help him set up his new religious congregation. Michael Rua was a most amazing young man, and Fr. John Bosco recognized this. More and more, Fr. John relied on Michael as his right-hand helper. Eventually, Michael Rua would come to be called "The Second Father of the Salesian Order." In 1855, Michael made his religious vows in this new congregation.

In the same year, Michael joined John Bosco in nursing the sick during a cholera epidemic that swept the city. Michael did his nursing, and also worked as a catechist, in the slums of Turin.

In 1860, Michael was ordained a priest, and from that time on, he was constantly at Fr. John Bosco's side. In 1865, Fr. Michael became the vicar of the Salesian Order.

Fr. Michael, in addition to his nursing and teaching duties, was an outstanding administrator. By the time Michael died, the congregation had grown to 4,000 Salesians in 345 communities, and was found in 33 nations of the world. Fr. Michael gained the nickname "the living rule" because of his great fidelity to St. John Bosco's vision for the Order.

Fr. Michael Rua died in on April 6, 1910 at the age of 72 in Turin.

Pope Paul VI beatified him on October 29, 1972.

Blessed Michael Rua's feast day is April 6.

81

Ven. Nicola D'Onofrio, M.I.
March 24, 1943 – June 12, 1964

NICOLA D'ONOFRIO WAS BORN ON March 24, 1943 in Villamagna, Chieti, Italy. His father was a farmer, and his mother was known for her piety and knowledge of her faith. It was Nicola's mother who raised Nicola to be a sensitive, compassionate, and peaceful person.

As a child, Nicola faithfully served Mass in his local parish church even in the dead of winter, and he distinguished himself as a very kind student, always available for others.

When he was around 12 years old, Nicola met a Camillian priest who invited him to enter the Camillian seminary to study to become a priest. His father objected because he needed him to work in the fields as a farmhand, and his mother objected because she wanted him to go to the diocesan seminary. Even his unmarried aunts tempted him to stay by promising him an inheritance.

Though Nicola did stay for a time, his parents finally gave in, and he was able to enter the Seminary of St. Camillus in Rome. He entered on October 3, 1955, which was at that time the feast day of St. Therese, the Little Flower, one of his favorite saints. Though there were many students in the seminary, the Camillian authorities could not help but notice this young man whose personality seemed to shine.

On October 6, 1960, Nicola received the habit of his Order, beginning his novitiate year. During this year, he learned about St. Camillus de Lellis (another Saintly Man of Nursing in this book) and about the Camillian tradition of care for the sick as nurses and other health professionals.

Nicola learned how to recognize Christ in patients and treat them accordingly. Once, for example, when he was nursing an older priest with throat cancer on Good Friday, he reminded the priest, "Father, unite your pains to those of Christ in agony, for today is Good Friday, a blessed day for you who suffer together with Jesus."

On October 7, 1961, the feast of Our Lady of the Rosary, Nicola made his first vows of poverty, chastity, obedience, and "charity towards the sick even in cases of contagious diseases."

As a young Religious, Nicola was found by his confreres to be a very diligent and peaceful young man, humble and always willing to do whatever needed to be done in the community. The future looked very bright indeed for this handsome young man who had found his calling.

At the end of 1962, however, Nicola began experiencing symptoms that would lead to a diagnosis of cancer in 1963.

When Nicola learned that his cancer was terminal, he accepted it with grace and serenity as God's will for him. He was not afraid to talk of his disease or its treatment, but neither did overly dramatize it.

Despite the bleak outlook for his physical health, Nicola was permitted to enroll at the Pontifical Gregorian University to begin philosophy studies.

Because of Nicola's illness, Pope Paul VI gave him special dispensation to take his final vows early. Therefore, on May 28, 1964, the feast of Corpus Christi, Nicola consecrated his life to God forever in the church at the Camillian seminary.

For the next several days, Nicola suffered almost insufferable pain. But he tried to hide his pain whenever possible, to avoid being a burden to those who were nursing him.

Nicola died on June 12, 1964 at the age of 21.

Pope Francis named Nicola as a Venerable on July 5, 2013.

Venerable Nicola D'Onofrio never had the opportunity to be ordained a priest, or to become a full-fledged nurse. However, he serves as a symbol of all men who never got the chance to become a nurse, either because of poverty or because nursing schools banned their admission because of their gender.

But Venerable Nicola is also a symbol of all people who have a dream and seek to fulfill that dream. Nicola's holy life shows that it is the journey to the dream that is important, for it is on the journey that one becomes a saint.

82

Bl. Oddino Barrotti, O.S.F.
1334 (or 1324) – July 7, 1400

ODDINO BARROTTI WAS BORN IN either 1324 or 1334 in Fossano, Piedmont, to a well-known Fossano family.

When he grew up, Oddino became a diocesan priest and was assigned to the parish of St. John the Baptist in his hometown.

It was not long before this priest became recognized for his great love for the poor and for the austere life he led. Sometimes, however, Fr. Oddino did not exercise prudence in his spiritual life: the bishop had to order him to eat meat once in a while and to keep some of the collection for the upkeep of the parish instead of giving it all away to the poor.

In 1374, Fr. Oddino was assigned as provost for a collegiate chapter of a pious confraternity in Fossano and rector of a parish. He faithfully served in these ministries until four years later when he resigned to become director of a religious community. At that time, he became a Franciscan tertiary and turned his house into a hospital. It was there that he probably got his first experience of nursing the sick.

In 1381, Fr. Oddino went on a pilgrimage to the Holy Land. Unfortunately, the Turks captured and imprisoned him for a short time. While in prison, he became known for working miracles.

When he returned to his home, he was appointed governor of the Guild of the Cross, a pious association for the care of the sick and hospitality to pilgrims.

Also at this time, Fr. Oddino built a hospital with an attached guesthouse. There he and his associates could not only nurse the sick, but also could show hospitality to pilgrims. This institution was said never to have turned away a pilgrim or a sick person. It lasted into the nineteenth century.

Because of Fr. Oddino's great ability as an organizer and builder, he was once asked by another priest to build a new church. He agreed to do this, and soon stories began to be told about him. People began saying that Fr. Oddino had superhuman strength, able to lift and move giant loads by himself. Others told that one day, a mason fell to his death while building the tower of the church; Fr. Oddino supposedly raised the man from the dead.

In 1400, plague devastated his town. Fr. Oddino immediately began nursing the sick and meeting their spiritual needs at the same time. Fr. Oddino caught the plague himself from his nursing, and died on July 7, 1400.

Pope Pius VII approved the title of "Blessed" for Oddino Barrotti in 1880.

Blessed Oddino Barrotti's feast day is July 7.

83

St. Paul of the Cross, C.P.
January 3, 1694 – October 18, 1775

PAULO FRANCESCO DANEI WAS BORN on January 3, 1694 in Piedmont, the second of sixteen children. Though his father had a dry goods store, the family was a poor one.

After receiving his early education from a priest who operated a school for boys in Cremolino, Lombardy, Paul left school and returned home. There, Paul taught catechism in various churches.

When he was around 19, Paul joined his father as a soldier. It did not take Paul long to realize that the life of a soldier did not suit him, so he returned home. On his journey home, however, he stopped at the town called of Novello, where he nursed an elderly couple until the end of 1716.

When he was 26 years old, Paul had three visions of starting a new religious order. When he sought advice from his bishop, the bishop told him his visions were real, and that he should go ahead to follow them.

With the bishop's good wishes, Paul spent 40 days in prayers and penance. During this retreat, Paul wrote a rule for a new order, which would eventually become known as the Congregation of the Passion of Jesus Christ, or simply the Passionists.

After Paul's retreat, his brother John Baptist and two other young men joined him. Besides the traditional vows of poverty, chastity and obedience, the men took a fourth vow to become devoted to the passion of Christ. By 1747, the new Order had three monasteries which they called "retreats." In

Religious life, Paul became "Paul of the Cross," the title by which he is known today.

Because Paul thought there would be better chances of getting his Order approved if the men lived in Rome, Paul and John Baptist took up residence there. There, at the invitation of Cardinal Corrandini, they established a new hospital and nursed the sick. They also provided pastoral care to the patients and the staff. So profound was his nursing care, that even during his lifetime, Paul was known as a miracle-worker and healer.

On June 7, 1727, Pope Benedict XIII ordained John Baptist and Paul. After ordination, the brothers began preaching throughout Italy.

Fr. Paul died on October 18, 1775. By that time, the Passionists had 180 priests and Brothers living in 12 Retreats.

Pope Blessed Pius IX canonized Paul on June 29, 1867.

The feast day of St. Paul of the Cross is October 20 in the United States.

84

St. Peter of St. Joseph de Betancur, O.F.B.
March 21, 1626 – April 25, 1667

PETER DE BETANCUR WAS BORN on March 21, 1626 in Vilaflor on Tenerife, the largest of the Canary Islands, as one of five children of a poor family.

As a child, Peter worked as a shepherd, caring for his family's small flock of sheep. He also loved to spend time praying in the solitude of a small cave.

In 1638, a moneylender demanded that Peter's father pay the family debt. Because the family was too poor to pay their debt, Peter was indentured to the moneylender.

When he was 23 years old, Peter became free from his service to the moneylender, whereupon he decided to leave the Canary Islands and sail to Guatemala. There, he hoped to connect with a relative who worked for the government.

By the time Peter reached Havana, however, he had no more money. Destitute, he worked for a year for a priest who was also from Tenerife. After the year was over, Peter paid for passage to Honduras by working as a crew-member of the ship. From Honduras, he walked to Guatemala.

When he got to Guatemala City, poor Peter was again destitute, and he found himself in a bread line sponsored by Franciscans.

Before long, Peter entered a Jesuit college to study for the priesthood. Unfortunately, probably because of a lack of a solid education in his formative years, Peter could not master the material and had to leave. He decided that God wanted him to serve him at least in the lay state, so in 1655, Peter became a lay Franciscan in Antigua, Guatemala. There, he took the name Peter of St. Joseph as his lay Franciscan name.

God showered many blessings on Peter, including energy, focused vision, and good administrative skills. Peter accepted these gifts and developed them.

First, he devoted himself to poor youth and to the destitute of society – prisoners, the sick, and the unemployed. In 1658, someone gave Peter a hut which he converted into a hospital for the poor who needed post-hospital care. There, he nursed them with love, compassion, and sensitivity. Soon, people began to hear about and admire his devotion to nursing. As a result, powerful people such as the bishop and governor began to support his efforts.

Within three years after turning his hut into a little hospital, benefactors provided Peter with land and workers to build him a larger hospital, thoroughly stocked and equipped. Now, he could nurse to his heart's content. Before long, Peter added a homeless shelter, a school for the poor, and an inn for priests. Peter put his work under the patronage of Our Lady of Bethlehem.

Like all good leaders, Peter attracted others to himself. Almost before he knew it, there appeared other Franciscan tertiaries that wanted to help him with his nursing and related work. He taught them nursing theory and skills so they could assist in the hospital. But soon, he created a Rule for the group based on the Rule of St. Augustine. Eventually, this group became a religious Order called the Bethlehemites, whose primary purpose was to serve the sick as nurses and related health care providers. In time, the Bethlehemites served in two other of the city's hospitals.

Women also adopted this rule and devoted themselves to teaching poor children.

Though Peter's first concern was nursing the sick, he also had a great love for prisoners and visited them frequently. Often at night he would wander the streets ringing a bell to remind people to pray, especially for the dead.

St. Peter of St. Joseph de Betancur has the honor of being the first saint of the Canary Islands, the first saint of Guatemala, and the first saint of Central America.

During his life, Peter was known as a miracle worker, frequently healing the sick almost immediately. Not surprisingly, miracles are continually being reported at his tomb and in the cave on Tenerife where he liked to spend time as a youth.

Many historians credit St. Peter as taking the pre-Christmas *posadas* custom to Central American nations as well as to Mexico. The *posadas* are nine days of celebration that runs from December 16 through 24, celebrating Joseph's and Mary's search for a *posada* – or inn - in Bethlehem.

Peter died on April 25, 1667 in Antigua, Guatemala.

Pope St. John Paul II canonized Peter in Guatemala City on July 30, 2002.

St. Peter of St. Joseph de Betancur is a patron saint of Guatemala, Guatemalan catechists, the Canary Islands, all of Central America, and the homeless, and he is an honorary mayor of various towns of Guatemala and the Canary Islands.

85

St. Peter Claver, S.J.
June 26, 1581 – September 8, 1654

PETER CLAVER WAS BORN ON June 26, 1581 in the Spanish village of Verdú to a prosperous farming family.

As a young man, he studied at the Jesuit-run University of Barcelona. In 1601, he entered the Jesuit Order and made first vows on August 7, 1602. In his further studies in Majorca, Peter came in contact with a man who would greatly influence the rest of his life – the college porter, St. Alphonsus Rodríguez. It was Alphonsus who inspired Peter to become a missionary to the New World.

In April of 1610, after Peter finished his theological studies in Barcelona, he was chosen to represent the Jesuit province of Aragon in an assembly of Jesuits going to what was then called "New Granada," today known as Colombia and Panama.

In April of 1610, Peter left Spain for the New World, never to return. He landed in Cartagena, in what is now Colombia. From there, he went to Bogotá to finish his theological studies. There he worked as a sacristan, porter, nurse, and cook. After doing his final year of Religious formation in Tunja, Peter returned to Cartagena in 1615 and was ordained a priest there on March 19, 1616.

As a newly ordained priest, Fr. Peter began his life's work: to serve the African slaves who were being brought to Cartagena, a major slave center at that time. Peter was horrified at the inhumane way the slaves were treated, and he was so determined to devote his entire life to making their life better, that he took a fourth vow: to be the "slave of the Africans."

Fortunately for Fr. Peter, he first served under the guidance of Jesuit Fr. Alfonso de Sandoval (who is also listed in this book as a Saintly Man of Nursing). Fr. Alfonso had worked with the slaves for over 40 years, and he had produced not only practical tips on how to help the slaves, but also much scholarly sociological and cultural anthropological ethnographic research.

For the next 40 years, Fr. Peter gave himself tirelessly to the care of the slaves. From his window in his rectory, he could view the arrival of new ships. Whenever he spotted a new ship in the port, he would dash out of his house to meet it. There, he would do everything he could to reduce the fears of the terrified slaves and nurse them.

Fr. Peter, though his main focus was the slaves, also gave pastoral care to prisoners, crewmembers, slave owners, and others. Peter also did nursing in the two hospitals of Cartagena. One of the hospitals was St. Sebastian, a general hospital run by the Brothers of St. John of God (another Saintly Man of Nursing in this book); the other was St. Lazarus Hospital for lepers and those suffering from St. Anthony's Fire (erysipelas).

Peter devoted many hours to preaching in the streets of Cartagena. It is easy to see why many began calling Fr. Peter, "the Apostle of Cartagena."

In his forty years, he instructed and baptized more than 300,000 people.

In 1650, when he was about 70, Peter went to preach to African slaves along the coast. Soon, however, he became sick and had to go back to Cartagena. He was the first of the Jesuits to catch the plague that was raging through the area, and he was close to death. For the next four years, Fr. Peter was basically confined to his room. Unfortunately, the person who was assigned to care for him was negligent, but Fr. Peter never complained at his lack of care. He recovered, but was never able to return to his ministries.

In 1654, Fr. Diego Ramírez-Farina arrived from Spain to continue Fr. Peter's work. Fr. Peter was so thrilled to hear the news that his loving work would continue among the African slaves, that he was able to rise from his bed to greet his successor.

Fr. Peter died on September 7 or 8, 1654. Though the civil and religious authorities of his time often criticized his work among the slaves as "displaced enthusiasm," they now competed with one another to give him honors. Peter was buried with a great ceremony, and Africans and Indians offered a second Mass in his honor.

Fr. Peter's amazing influence spread throughout the world.

On January 15, 1888, Pope Leo XIII canonized Peter along with his mentor, Alphonsus Rodríguez.

St. Peter Claver's feast day is September 9. He is a patron saint of all missionary activities among black-skinned peoples.

86

Bl. Peter Donders, C.Ss.R.
October 27, 1809 – January 14, 1887

PETER DONDERS WAS BORN IN Tilburg, Netherlands on October 27, 1809 to a poor couple. Because of the family's poverty, Peter and his brother Martin had to help support the family financially. Therefore, they had to leave school at a young age to work.

Because Peter wanted to be a priest but did not have money for the seminary, his parish priest convinced the officials at the minor seminary to take him in as a servant, and to let him study in his leisure time. The officials agreed, and Peter went to work as a servant and, on the side, a seminarian.

When he was 26, Peter was ready to enter the major seminary. His advisors convinced him to apply to a religious order, perhaps to secure funds for tuition. Peter applied to the Jesuits, Redemptorists, and Franciscans, but all of these Orders refused his admission.

Somehow, Peter was ordained a diocesan priest in 1841.

The following year, he decided to be a foreign missionary in Suriname, which was then a Dutch colony in South America. (Today, Suriname is the smallest nation in South America.)

Fr. Peter was to spend the rest of his life serving the people in this part of the world. From 1842 to 1866, he served as a diocesan priest, and from 1866 to his death in 1887 he served as a Redemptorist priest.

In the first 14 years in Suriname, Fr. Peter did parish ministry in the capital city of Paramaribo. This involved the usual duties of a parish priest –

celebrating Mass, visiting the sick, administering the sacraments, counseling, writing, conducting funerals and burying the dead, and a host of others.

In 1856, Fr. Peter volunteered to go to the leper colony of Batavia. There he spent his time nursing the lepers and teaching people about their Faith. Eventually he was able to persuade authorities to send more nurses to help him in his work and improve the dismal conditions under which the lepers lived.

In 1865, the Vatican put Suriname under the care of the Redemptorist Order. The following year, the Redemptorist Fathers accepted Fr. Peter and another priest as novices in the Order. In June of 1867, when they had finished their novitiate year, the two men became Redemptorist priests.

Soon, Fr. Peter was back with the lepers he loved so much. This time, however, there was another priest to help. Now that he had some help, he decided to carry the Faith to the indigenous peoples – Caribs, Arrowaks, and Warros – and to runaway slaves living in the forests.

The missionary travels to primitive regions were often very dangerous, but this never stopped Fr. Peter from his mission. Fr. Peter spent the rest of his life caring for the lepers and indigenous peoples for the rest of his life, taking only one short break in Batavia.

Fr. Peter died on January 14, 1887 and was buried in the leper cemetery.
Pope St. John Paul II beatified Fr. Peter on May 23, 1982.
Blessed Peter Donders' feast day is January 14.

87

Bl. Peter Tecelano, O.F.S.
c. 1200 – December 1289

PETER TECELANO WAS BORN IN Campi, Tuscany around 1200. When he was a child, his family moved from Campi to Siena.

When he grew up, Peter got married and worked as a comb-maker in his town. Pietro and his wife had a happy life together until she died. The couple never had children.

After the death of his wife, Peter began working in a Franciscan hospital – Santa Maria della Scala - as a nurse. Attracted to the Franciscans, he became a member of the Third Order of St. Francis. While nursing, he also continued his comb-making business. From the money he made, he gave much of it to the Franciscans for their good works. During this time, Peter led a very simple and solitary life. At night, he could often be found in the local church praying.

Through his prayer and meditation, Peter decided that he wanted to live a life more closely connected to the Franciscans. Fortunately, the Franciscans, who ran the local hospital, agreed to allow Peter to live in a cell of the monastery closest to the infirmary. While he lived in this cell, Peter would frequently visit the sick and dedicate himself to prayer.

Soon, Peter began to be known throughout Siena as a miracle worker and a mystic. Not surprisingly, therefore, many laypersons and priests chose him as their spiritual advisor.

While living at the monastery, Peter was always trying to improve himself. His biggest fault, from his perspective, was being too talkative. Therefore, he tried to foster silence in his life as much as it was prudently possible.

Peter died in early December of 1289.

Soon after Peter's death, people began flocking to his grave where miracles were frequently reported.

Many people believe that the poet, Dante Alighieri, based the character "Pier the Comb-Seller" in his *Divine Comedy* on Blessed Peter Tecelano.

Blessed Peter of Siena's feast day is December 10th.

88

St. Philip Neri, C.O.
July 21, 1515 – May 25 or 26, 1595

PHILIP NERI WAS BORN ON July 21, 1515 in Florence. His father was in the legal profession, and his mother was of noble background. As a child, he received an excellent education at a Dominican school in Florence.

When he was 18, Philip's father sent him to live with his uncle, Romolo, a wealthy merchant in San Germano, not only to assist him in business, but to learn as much as possible about becoming a merchant himself.

While he was in San Germano, Philip frequently visited the monks of Monte Cassino. In his visits, he learned that he was attracted to Catholic liturgy, community life, and solitude. After a year with his uncle, Philip had a religious experience that turned him from worldly pursuits to more spiritual ones. With this new awakening, Philip went to Rome in 1533.

Rome, following its sacking in 1527 by the Holy Roman Emperor, was in a sorry state. Many of its churches had been desecrated, and many works of art had been destroyed. In this context, Philip took up lodging in the house of a customs agent. To earn his keep, he tutored the man's two sons. He lived extremely frugally, living on bread, olives, wine and water.

While in Rome, Philip began studying philosophy and theology. He also found himself drawn to nursing the sick and caring for the poor and the prostitutes of Rome. Philip served as a lay missionary of sorts in Rome. Around 1544, he met St. Ignatius of Loyola who had just established the Society of Jesus (Jesuits). It was at this time that Philip had a mystical experience that determined the rest of his life. The experience that Philip had was of the Spirit entering his body causing severe heart palpitations.

Because of his great work in Rome, people began calling Philip "the apostle of Rome." Soon, other men began to be attracted to him, and in 1548 he founded the *Confraternity of the Most Holy Trinity of Pilgrims and Convalescents*. The purposes of this group of men were to minister to the thousands of pilgrims who visited Rome, and to nurse patients who had been discharged from hospitals but were not quite ready to be on their own. This group prayed together, worked together, and celebrated Forty Hours Devotion together frequently.

On May 23, 1551, Philip was ordained a priest on the advice of his spiritual director. Fr. Philip had many saintly friends including St. Ignatius of Loyola, St. Francis Xavier, and St. Camillus de Lellis. (Both St. Francis Xavier and St. Camillus are Saintly Men of Nursing in this book.)

After his ordination, Fr. Philip nursed the sick at San Giacomo Hospital. Soon other men sought him out and wanted to help. Philip, who was known for his cheerful and loving nature, attracted others like him. Soon, they began to meet for prayer, Bible study, and work. In time, the group became a religious community known as the Oratory, whose members were called Oratorians.

In Philip's vision, Oratorians were all equal, and all were expected to pull their weight. The wealthy, for example, were expected to nurse the sick and beg for alms just as others.

Though Fr. Philip did nursing and other tasks to help society, his special gift was as a confessor.

Fr. Philip was active to the very end of his life, celebrating Mass, preaching, and hearing confessions. He died on the morning of May 25 or 26, 1591.

Pope Gregory XV canonized him on March 12, 1622.

St. Philip Neri's feast day is May 26.

St. Philip Neri is a patron saint of laughter, humor, joy, Rome and many other cities.

89

Bl. Pier Giorgio Frassati, T.O.S.D.
April 6, 1901 – July 4, 1925

PIER GIORGIO FRASSATI WAS BORN in Turin, Italy, on April 6, 1901. His father was an agnostic who owned a progressive newspaper called *La Stampa*. In later life, Pier's father was an Italian senator and ambassador to Germany. Unlike his agnostic father, Pier's mother was a devout Catholic Christian.

From a very young age, Pier had a great devotion to the poor and the sick, and was deeply devoted to Catholic social teaching. Pier was especially influenced by Pope Leo XIII's encyclical, *Rerum Novarum* – "Rights and Duties of Capital and Labor." This encyclical was the Catholic answer to the Industrial Revolution, a time when men were torn from their homes to work for industrial giants that often mistreated them. *Rerum Novarum* insisted on various rights of workers, the duties of management, and the concept of the preferential option for the poor, that is, Jesus' teaching that marginalized people have the greatest moral claim on Christians' consciences.

Pier frequently said, "Charity is not enough; we need social reform." He often preached social action to his fellow students, and he was active in various groups of Catholic students who wanted a better society. Pier was passionately against right-wing political movements such as fascism. Although Pier had a very playful nature and loved to engage in the arts and mountain hiking, he was no stranger to political rallies that condemned right-wing political ideologies.

Pier was also attracted to various Dominican saints, and he became a member of the Third Order of St. Dominic. He was especially attracted to the Dominican friar, Girolamo Savonarola, an excommunicated firebrand Church reformer of the fifteenth century. He even adopted Girolamo's first name as his own at times.

But Pier did not merely talk about Catholic social justice. Rather, he devoted his short life to practicing it. For example, even though his family was very wealthy, Pier's father did not want his children to be spoiled. Thus, he gave Pier and his sister Luciana only a little money to spend. Pier was notoriously known for giving his money away to people he regarded as more needy than himself. Frequently, he would have to run all the way home because he had given away his train fare. Often, he would travel in the poorest section of the train so he could give extra money to the poor. Once, when his friends asked him why he was traveling in third class of the train, he replied with a smile, "Because there is no fourth class."

Because Pier always tried to do his good deeds in secret, his nursing activities were not well known until after his death. But we know that Pier would often not come home at night because he was in hospitals nursing poor people who were unwell. And we know he made nursing rounds in individual homes of the poor, for on his deathbed, he stipulated that medicine be delivered to one of his patients.

Pier's sister, Luciana, writes in *A Man of the Beatitudes: Pier Giorgio Frassati,*

> He had a great love for the sick, from whom one day he would contact the fatal polio. It was among the sick that he had found the best opportunity to share his humanity, and it was among the sick that he reached the end of his human pilgrimage.

Pier, shares two traits with many other Saintly Men of Nursing. First, like many saintly nurses, it was through nursing the sick that he found the body of Christ in a very concrete way. And second, like so many other nurses, a disease he picked up from nursing the sick killed him.

Pier died from poliomyelitis on July 4, 1925 at the age of 24. Because Pier's father held important government positions, Pier's family expected Turin's political and social elite to pay their respects. They were shocked, however, to discover the streets of Turin lined with thousands of ordinary people as Nicola's cortege passed by.

The Pier Giorgio Frassati College of Nursing is located in Suryapet, India. The Catholic Diocese of Nalgonda runs the college.

On May 20, 1990, Pope St. John Paul II beatified Pier.

Blessed Pier Giorgio Frassati's feast day is July 4.

90

Bl. Raphael Chylinski, O.F.M. Conv.
January 8, 1694 – December 2, 1741

MELCHOIR CHYLINSKI WAS BORN ON January 8, 1694 in Pozman, Poland to an aristocratic family. His parents were devout Catholic Christians, and they instilled a love of their faith in Melchoir.

From a very early age, Melchoir wanted to be a priest. It was no surprise, then, at the age of 21, April 4, 1714, Melchoir entered the Conventual Franciscans Order in Cracow, and was given the new name, Raphael.

Raphael was ordained a priest in 1717. After ordination, he went for further studies in Warsaw and Lagiewnicki (near Lodz). In his priesthood, he served in various Conventual Franciscan communities and various parishes.

Fr. Raphael became a priest in what historians often call the "Dark Ages of Poland." At that time, Poland had just finished the Thirty Years War and the population was exhausted. The rich were indifferent and demoralized, and there was widespread poverty in the land. The country, as always, was worried about invasions from their neighbors, and the Catholic Church was fearful of Protestant and Orthodox influence in Poland.

Fr. Raphael became well known not only as a man of prayer, but also as one who frequently gave his meager food rations and few clothes to the sick and the poor.

In 1734, Russia invaded Poland, leading to a host of: famine, civil disorder, battles, blockades of goods, and epidemics.

It was during this time that a severe epidemic came to Warsaw. Fr. Raphael, without hesitation or concern for his own safety, began nursing the sick, caring for mind, body, and spirit.

Fr. Raphael died on December 2, 1741.

Pope St. John Paul II beatified him on June 9, 1991.

Blessed Raphael Chylinski's feast day is December 2.

91

Bl. Raymond of Capua, O.P.
c. 1330 – October 5, 1399

RAYMOND DELLE VIGNA WAS BORN around 1330 in Capua, Kingdom of Naples, to a prominent family.

In 1350, while he was studying law at the University of Bologna, Raymond entered the Dominican Order. After ordination, Fr. Raymond worked in many Dominican friaries in Italy including Rome, Florence, and Siena. Most of his work involved spiritual direction and administration.

While in Siena, Fr. Raymond made friends with the great saint, Catherine of Siena, who was a Dominican tertiary. Raymond and Catherine became close friends, and Raymond became her advisor.

In 1374, a plague came to Siena, and Fr. Raymond began to nurse the sick. Unfortunately, through his nursing, Fr. Raymond caught the plague himself. As he lay near death, Catherine stayed at his bedside, praying for him and nursing him until he recovered. Raymond attributed his recovery to Catherine's prayers.

Beside nursing, spiritual direction, and administration, Fr. Raymond also actively made his views known in the papal intrigues of his time and reforming the Dominican Order. He and Catherine were both on the same side in the "Great Western Schism" that found different men claiming to be pope.

In 1380, Catherine of Siena died, and in the same year, Fr. Raymond became the Master General of the Dominican Order. Because of his reforms and great administrative achievements, he is sometimes called the "second founder of the Order of Preachers."

Fr. Raymond was also a writer, producing biographies of St. Catherine of Siena and St. Agnes of Montepulciano.

While advocating for reform of his Order in Germany, Fr. Raymond died on October 5, 1399 in Nuremberg.

Pope Leo XIII beatified Raymond on the fifth century of his death in 1899.

Blessed Raymond of Capua's feast day is October 5.

92

St. Rock

c. 1348 – c. 1376

IN THE MORE THAN 2,000 years of Catholic Christianity, many legends have been told about holy people. Because the legends are shrouded by mystery and cannot be verified, they stand as interesting stories that may or may not be true. Or, better yet, they may have elements that are true but have been embellished so much that no one knows where fact ends and myth begins. In many such cases, as in all myths, the lessons to be learned are genuine even if the facts are questionable. Such is the case of St. Rock – also known as Roch, Rocco, Roque, and others.

One of the most common biographies of Rock says he was born in Montpellier, France around 1348 to the governor of Montpellier and his wife. At the age of 20, after both of his parents had died, he went to Rome on a pilgrimage. In Italy at that time there occurred an epidemic, perhaps of the plague, and Rock found himself nursing the sick not only in Rome, but also in Acquapendene, Cesena, Rimini, and Novara. In his legend, Rock cured many people simply by making the Sign of the Cross over them.

While at Piacenza, Rock became infected by the plague himself. Because he didn't want to burden the hospital, he took himself out to the woods to die. Fortunately, however, a dog found him and brought him bread to eat every day. Eventually, the dog's master found Rock and nursed him back to health.

After he was cured, Rock went back to Piacenza to nurse the sick, and cured many. It was there that he began nursing and curing cattle as well as people.

Eventually Rock returned to Montpellier. Unfortunately, his uncle did not recognize Rock and had him imprisoned for five years on a charge of spying. After Rock died in prison, a cross-shaped birthmark on his breast was revealed. Only then did his family and friends recognize that this man was Rock, the former governor's son. As a result of the discovery, he was given a public funeral. Many miracles were attributed to Rock in death, just as they had been attributed to him when he was alive.

Rock was declared a saint by "popular fervor," and Pope Gregory XIV added his name to the *Roman Martyrology* around 1590.

St. Rock's fame spread throughout Europe, and in many rural areas, people bring their cattle for blessing on his feast day. Legend also has it that there was once a man who doubted the divine origin of wheat, so God destroyed the entire harvest with a terrible storm. St. Rock prayed, "Dear God, let me have a little wheat, just enough to grind for my dog." Many people continue to say this prayer for an abundant harvest.

St. Rock's feast day is August 16.

St. Rock is a patron saint of people with diseases such as plague and cholera; bachelors; diseased cattle and dogs; falsely accused people; invalids; surgeons; tile makers; gravediggers; second-hand dealers, pharmacists; and the cities of Potenza and Girifalco in Italy and of Istanbul in Turkey.

93

St. Salvius of Albi, O.S.B.
d. 584

WHAT IS KNOWN ABOUT SALVIUS comes from reports from his friend, St. Gregory of Tours. Though we don't know the date of his birth, Gregory says Salvius was born in Albi in what is now known as France.

Trained as a lawyer, he served for a time as a judge. Salvius never married, and during the time he practiced law, he lived with his mother.

One day, however, Salvius gave up his legal career and joined a monastery on the outskirts of Albi. He loved solitude, and even he admitted that he often practiced austerities to excess.

The other monks elected him as their abbot, but he continued living more as a hermit than a monk. Though he lived a solitary life, his door was always open to monks or others who wished to see him. One time he became violently ill from a fever, but he recovered. Stories began circulating that he had died and was restored to health.

In 547, Salvius was consecrated Bishop of Albi. Despite this honor, he continued to live his life as austerely as ever. Any money or material goods that people gave him as bishop, he would promptly give away to the poor.

While Salvius was bishop, the two biggest problems he encountered in his diocese were Arianism and paganism. Arianism denied the divinity of Jesus, while in Salvius' time, "pagan" referred to anyone who did not believe in God.

Despite Salvius' love of solitude and reputation as a hermit, he had excellent social skills that allowed him to reconcile interpersonal conflicts.

In 584, an epidemic of some sort raged through Albi. Despite his friends' pleas not to be in contact with the victims, Bishop Salvius insisted on personally nursing the sick. Not only did he nurse the infected patients, he also prepared them for death and consoled their families.

Because of his nursing, Salvius became infected himself. When he realized he would die of the disease, which many believe was plague, he ordered a casket to be made for him, changed his clothes, and was ready for his death on September 10, 584.

Many churches of his time were named after him.

St. Salvius of Albi's feast day is September 10.

94

Bl. Samuel Marzorati, O.F.M.
September 10, 1670 – March 3, 1716

ANTONIO FRANCESCO MARZORATI WAS BORN on September 10, 1670 in Biumo Inferiore, Varese, Lombardy.

On March 5, 1692, Antonio joined the Franciscan Order in Lugano, Switzerland, took the name Samuel, and was ordained to the priesthood.

Because Fr. Samuel asked to become a foreign missionary, his superiors sent him to study at St. Peter's College in Montorio, Italy. After completing his studies and serving at another task, Fr. Samuel was given orders to go to Ethiopia.

In autumn of 1711, Fr. Samuel joined two other Franciscan priests, Fathers Liberatus and Michael Pius, both of whom are also Saintly Men of Nursing in this book. The two priests had suffered immensely in Ethiopia, and they had to flee to Egypt. Fathers Liberatus and Michael Pius were the only two men left of their original group of eight priests and three lay brothers sent by the Society for the Propagation of the Faith to Ethiopia.

Fr. Liberatus, who was the superior of the delegation, led his two fellow friars to Ethiopia. They landed at Massawa on April 18, 1712 after a very difficult journey, and then they made their way to Gonder, which was the capital at that time. They arrived there in July 1712.

Though the ruler, Justos, welcomed them, he could not allow them to preach because of his precarious hold on power and the anti-Christian sentiment of the country.

To make the best use of their time, Fr. Samuel and his companions learned the language and customs of the people and opened a hospital. There they nursed the sick for free.

Three years after the three friars arrived in Ethiopia, malicious rumors began to be spread about them. At about the same time, Justos was forced to abdicate, and his successor was a young and inexperienced man named David III.

Samuel, Liberatus, and Michael were sentenced to death by stoning because of their faith. The night before their martyrdom, they spent all night singing songs of praise to God.

Samuel and his companions were taken in chains to Abbo, the place of execution, and were stoned to death by a mob on March 3, 1716.

Pope St. John Paul II beatified Samuel and his companions on November 20, 1988.

The feast day of Blessed Samuel Marzorati and his two companions is March 3.

95

St. Simon of Lipnicza, O.F.M.
c. 1435 – July 18, 1482

SIMON WAS BORN SOMETIME BETWEEN 1435 and 1440 in Lipnicza Murowana, Poland.

From a very early age, Simon was known for his piety, especially his veneration of St. Mary. His parents ensured that he get a solid education not only in secular fields, but also in his Catholic Christian faith.

In 1454, Simon moved to Cracow to attend the University of Cracow. While there, he heard St. John of Capistrano speak about the Franciscan order. Therefore, in 1457, Simon and ten other university students were received into the Franciscan house at Stradom.

Simon was ordained a priest around 1460. He soon became famous as a very gifted preacher. In fact, he became the first Franciscan to be the official preacher at the Cathedral of Wawel, home of Poland's monarchy, in 1463. Before his appointment, only Dominicans served in this royal post.

Fr. Simon's preaching was very clear, especially in explaining the Bible. He also was very skilled at handing difficult and controversial topics. As a result, Fr. Simon converted many people to the Faith.

In 1478, Fr. Simon was pointed the *definitor* (advisor) of his Order in Cracow. After attending his Order's General Chapter, he traveled to the Holy Land hoping to perhaps be given the honor of being a martyr at the hands of the Turks. He did not receive that honor.

In 1482, after Fr. Simon returned to Cracow, plague struck the city. Fr. Simon and his colleagues devoted themselves to nursing the sick. From his nursing, Simon contracted the plague himself. As he lay dying, Simon asked that he be buried under the entrance of the church so that people entering the church would walk over his remains.

Fr. Simon died on July 18, 1482.

Pope Benedict XVI canonized him on June 3, 2007.

St. Simon of Lipnicza's feast day is July 18.

96

Ven. Simon Srugi, S.D.B.
June 27, 1877 – November 27, 1943

SIMON SRUGI WAS BORN ON June 27, 1877 in Nazareth, the youngest of ten children. When he was three years old, his parents died and he went to live with his grandmother. At eleven, he went to live in an orphanage in Bethlehem, which was run by the Salesian Fathers.

Simon loved the orphanage so much that when he was sixteen years old, he asked to be become a Salesian. The Order sent him to the Oratory Agricultural School at Beit Gemal. When he was finished with his studies, he became a Salesian Brother.

Brother Simon lived and worked in Beit Gemal for the rest of his life – fifty years. In Beit Gemal, Simon did many jobs at the Oratory such as porter, teacher, and storekeeper of a food and knickknack shop. What he was most famous for, however, was being the community nurse.

The mill at the Oratory was the only one in the area, so many farmers and their families had to come to the Oratory. People with ailments fell in love with the infirmarian and put all their trust in him. Even when there was a physician present, the people insisted on seeing Brother Simon. In fact, Muslims who came to the Oratory liked to say, "After Allah there was Srugi." They also said that Brother Simon was like a "cupful of honey."

Not only did Brother Simon treat his patients for various physical and psychosocial issues, he also blessed their children and served as peacemaker for people involved in various life dramas.

In 1908, Fr. Michael Rua – who is another Saintly Man of Nursing in this book and often called the "Second Father of the Salesian Order" – visited Beit Gemal. After observing Brother Simon, he told the community to "Follow him up well, record his words and deeds, because we are dealing here with a saint."

Brother Simon died from malaria on November 27, 1943 at the age of 66. Pope St. John Paul II declared Simon Venerable on April 2, 1993.

97

Bl. Stephen Bellesini, O.S.A.
November 25, 1774 – February 2, 1840

LUIGI GIUSEPPE BELLESINI WAS BORN on November 25, 1774 in Trent, in the Trentino region of what is now northern Italy.

When he was 16 years old, Luigi entered the Order of Hermits of St. Augustine and took the name of Stephen. Stephen was ordained a priest in 1797.

He studied in both Rome and Bologna, but had to return to Trent when Napoleon Bonaparte annexed various Papal States.

Fr. Stephen lived in his brother's house at this time and worked as a diocesan priest. During this time, he devoted himself to teaching children the Faith and to preaching. He was so successful in teaching, in fact, that the government made him the inspector of all the public schools in the Trentino region.

When the Papal States were once again restored, Fr. Stephen went back to Bologna, despite government opposition, to rejoin his Augustinian community. In his Order, he served as Novice Master, first in Rome, and then in Citta della Pieve. He then became the parish priest of the Augustinian church in Gennazzano, southeast of Rome. This church was famous for housing the icon of Our Lady of Good Counsel.

In 1839, a cholera epidemic devastated the area. It was during this epidemic, that Fr. Stephen fearlessly began nursing the sick. Unfortunately, from his nursing, he caught the disease himself and died on February 2, 1840.

Pope St. Pius X beatified Stephen on December 27, 1904.

Blessed Stephen Bellesini's feast day is February 3.

98

St. Toribio Romo-González
April 16, 1900 – February 25, 1928

TORIBIO ROMO-GONZÁLEZ WAS BORN ON April 16, 1900 on a ranch in Santa Ana de Guadalupe, Municipality of Jalostotitlán, in the State of Jalisco, Mexico. His humble parents raised him as a devout Catholic Christian, and Toribio was a conscientious altar server as a child.

When he was 13, Toribio began studying for the priesthood in the minor seminary at San Juan de los Lagos, and when he was 19, he entered the major seminary in Guadalajara. He was ordained a priest on December 23, 1922.

When Fr. Romo was ordained, the seeds of the Cristero War were sprouting. At this time the Mexican government was very anti-Catholic, and being a Catholic priest was quite dangerous. His first few years of priesthood were nomadic, as he and his companion priests had to move from one place to another for safety. Fr. Romo was noted for his great devotion to the Eucharist and to catechesis.

In 1927, Toribio's bishop asked him to be the parish priest in Tequila. Several other priests had earlier refused that assignment because it was in an extremely anti-Catholic area: being the parish priest of Tequila would be like signing one's own death warrant. Fr. Toribio Romo, however, did not hesitate to take the assignment.

When Fr. Romo got to Tequila, he learned that indeed the civil and military authorities in Tequila hated priests very much. Therefore, he stayed out of the main town and set up his headquarters in an abandoned tequila factory near a ranch called *"Agua Caliente,"* which ironically means "hot water" in English. There he taught religious classes to the people and celebrated Mass and other sacraments. This place was hidden by heavy vegetation. At night, under the cover of darkness, Fr. Toribio would secretly sneak into the town of Tequila to celebrate the Sacrament of the Sick and provide nursing care to those who were homebound.

At 5 a.m. on Saturday, February 25, 1928, federal officials broke into Toribio's room and shot him many times. His sister, Maria, was with him as he died. Like other Cristeros who fought against the anti-Catholic government, she exclaimed, "*Viva Cristo Rey*!" which means, "Long live Christ the King!"

The officials stripped Toribio naked while singing vulgar songs. They dragged his bloody body to the town and threw it in front of the town's courthouse. There, a powerful family claimed his body and prepared it for burial. The townspeople, in loving memory of their heroic priest, made a plaque that said, "The good shepherd lays down his life for his sheep."

Pope St. John Paul II canonized Fr. Toribio Romo González with other Mexican martyrs on May 21, 2000.

Now, although the story of St. Toribio Romo is amazing and inspirational in and of itself, it does not end at his death. In fact, Toribio's after-death nursing adventures are reportedly continuing even today in the deserts of Mexico and the United States in astonishing ways.

Today St. Toribio is the hero of legends and ballads resulting from his many mysterious appearances to immigrants coming from Mexico through the Sonoran Desert to the United States of America.

Many immigrants tell stories of being lost in the desert when suddenly a young priest appeared to them. In these experiences the priest nurses them by giving them food, drink, and a little money, and then guides them on their journey to the United States. In other words, he does what nurses have done for ages: he does for others what they cannot do for themselves. He tells them that if they ever return to Mexico, they should go to the town of Santa Ana de Guadalupe and ask for Toribio Romo. Those who have returned have been astonished when they got to the little church of Santa Ana de Guadalupe, for there in the church, they see a photo of the priest who appeared to them in the desert, St. Toribio Romo González. Many people call St. Toribio *"El Santo Coyote"* – The Holy Coyote.

Today thousands upon thousands of people journey to the tiny town of Santa Ana de Guadalupe, Jalisco to visit the shrine of St. Toribio Romo. They come to ask St. Toribio to help loved ones who are crossing the harsh desert to find a new life. Many of them have objects blessed to take with them on their journey. St. Toribio, who appears to be practicing nursing even today, is an unofficial patron saint of Mexican immigrants.

Pope John Paul II canonized Toribio on May 21, 2000.

St. Toribio Romo's feast day is May 21.

99

Bl. Vivaldo Stricchi, O.S.F.
1260 – May 1, 1320

VIVALDO STRICCHI, ALSO KNOWN AS Waldo, was born sometime in 1260 in San Gimignano, Tuscany to a wealthy family.

Unfortunately for Vivaldo, he and his friends became poor because of partying and wasting their money.

Having hit bottom, Vivaldo turned to a holy priest named Bartolo. Soon, they developed a great love for each other. When Fr. Bartolo contracted leprosy, Vivaldo determined to nurse him for the rest of Fr. Bartolo's life. And indeed, that is exactly what Vivaldo did. He nursed his friend for twenty years until Fr. Bartolo died in 1300.

During the time Vivaldo nursed his friend, he learned much about the spiritual life from Fr. Bartolo. At Fr. Bartolo's suggestion, Vivaldo joined the secular Franciscans.

After Fr. Bartolo died, Vivaldo decided to become a hermit. He found a large hollow chestnut tree where he made his hermitage. There, in this tiny space, Vivaldo lived for the next twenty years, praising God.

Legend has it that on May 1, 1320, bells from a church in a village near Vivaldo's hermitage began ringing on their own. Shortly thereafter, a hunter came to the village to report that his dogs had been circling an old chestnut tree, barking loudly. When the hunter approached the chestnut tree, he found Vivaldo dead in the cavity of the tree, in a kneeling position. As soon as the hunter finished his story, the bells of the church stopped ringing.

The residents of the village were convinced that the hermit was indeed a very holy man. They therefore brought his body back to the church and laid it to rest beneath the high altar. As years went by, many miracles began to be reported at the tomb of Waldo, and the people turned his chestnut tree cell into a chapel of St. Mary.

Blessed Vivaldo's feast day is May 1.

100

St. Zygmunt Gorazdowski
November 1, 1845 – January 1, 1920

ZYGMUNT GORAZDOWSKI WAS BORN ON November 1, 1845 in Sanok, Austrian Empire (today Poland) to a devout Catholic Christian family.

When Zygmunt was born, the area was experiencing great social-political turmoil. In an anti-serfdom event called the Galician Massacre of 1846, Zygmunt's nurse hid him under a mill wheel for his protection. This left him with a lung ailment, and Zygmunt required intensive therapy for this condition. On the bright side, his lifelong lung problems helped him develop a great sensitivity toward the sick. This sensitivity would last him all through his adult life.

When he was 18 years old, Zygmunt took part in the unsuccessful January Uprising against Russian occupation. When that movement failed, Zygmunt went to law school in what is now called Lviv, Ukraine, at that time under Austrian rule as part of the Habsburg Empire. After two years, however, he left law and entered the seminary.

Zygmunt was ordained a diocesan priest in 1871 and spent the next five to six years as an associate in various parishes. It was during this time that a cholera epidemic hit the area in which he lived, and Fr. Zygmunt became a hero through his nursing efforts. Not only did he nurse the sick without regard to his own personal safety, he also helped with preparing bodies after death.

In 1877, Fr. Zygmunt was assigned to the parish of St. Nicholas in Lviv, and in that town he worked for the next forty years.

In addition to caring for his parishioners, Fr. Zygmunt devoted much of his energy to helping the poor and the ill. For example, he founded soup kitchens, a health care center for the terminally ill and those needing convalescence, an institute for poor seminarians, a home for single mothers, an orphanage, and a Catholic school.

Because Fr. Zygmunt's many charities could not exist without the work of others, he founded the Religious Congregation of the Sisters of St. Joseph in 1884.

Fr. Zygmunt Gorazdowski died in Lviv on New Year's Day, 1920 at the age of 74. Many people who knew Fr. Zygmunt called him the "father of the poor and priest of the homeless."

Pope Benedict XVI canonized him on October 23, 2005.

St. Zygmunt's feast day is January 1.

Selected Bibliography

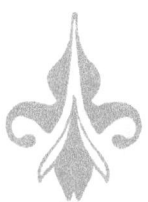

SELECTED BIBLIOGRAPHY

THE PURPOSE OF THIS SELECTED Bibliography is to provide a starting place for persons interested in learning more about these saintly men of nursing. It is not meant to be a comprehensive bibliography.

1 - Saint Aimo
- "St. Aimo," *Catholic Online/Saints & Angels*, no date.
- Contributors to Wikipedia. "Aimo." *Wikipedia: The Free Encyclopedia*, 24 April 2016.

2 - Saint Alonso de Sandoval
- Beers, M.E. "Alonso de Sandoval: Seventeenth-Century Merchant of the Gospel," World Wide Web, no date.

3 - Saint Aloysius Gonzaga
- "St. Aloysius Gonzaga." *Butler's Lives of the Saints: New Full Edition:*
- *June*, Revised by Kathleen Jones. Collegeville, MN: Burns & Oates/The Liturgical Press, 1997, pp. 152-156.
- "St. Aloysius Gonzaga." *Catholic Online/Saint of the Day*, no date.
- Contributors to Wikipedia. "Aloysius Gonzaga." *Wikipedia: The Free Encyclopedia*, 10 May 2017.

4 - Venerable Andrew Beltrami
- "Ven. Andrew Beltrami." *Salesian Missions online*, no date.

5 - Saint André Bessett
- "St. André Bessette (1845-1937) Porter, College Notre-Dame du Sacré-Coeur." EWTN, no date.
- "Blessed André Bessett." *Catholic Online/Saint of the Day*, no date.

- Contributors to Wikipedia. "André Bessette, C.S.C." *Wikipedia: The Free Encyclopedia*, 13 May 2017.

6 - Saint Anthelm
- "St. Anthelm." *Butler's Lives of the Saints: New Full Edition: April*, Revised by Peter Doyle. Collegeville, MN: Burns & Oates/The Liturgical press, 1999, pp. 200-202.
- "St. Anthelm." *Catholic Online/Saints & Angels*, no date.
- Contributors to Wikipedia. "Anthelm of Belley." *Wikipedia: The Free Encyclopedia*, 11 March 2017.

7 - Blessed Anthony Manzi
- "Blessed Anthony the Pilgrim." *Butler's Lives of the Saints: New Full Edition:*
- *February*, Revised by Paul Burns. Collegeville, MN: Burns & Oates/The Liturgical press, 1998, p. 8.
- "Bl. Anthony Manzi." *Catholic Online/Saints & Angels*, no date.
- "Blessed Anthony Manzi." *CatholicSaints.Info*, 29 January 2010. Web. 25 December 2015.

8 - Saint Anthony Mary Pucci
- "St. Anthony Mary Pucci." *Butler's Lives of the Saints: New Full Edition:*
- *January*, Revised by Paul Burns. Collegeville, MN: Burns & Oates/The Liturgical press, 1995, p. 86.
- "St. Anthony Mary Pucci." *Catholic Online/Saints & Angels*, no date.
- Contributors to Wikipedia. "Antonio Maria Pucci." *Wikipedia: The Free Encyclopedia*, 30 March 2017.

9 - Blessed Arnold Reche
- "Blessed Arnold Reche." *LaSalle.org*, no date.
- "Bl. Arnold Reche." *Butler's Lives of the Saints: New Full Edition:*
- *October*, Revised by Peter Boyle. Collegeville, MN: Burns & Oates/The Liturgical press, 1997, pp. 162-163.
- "Blessed Arnold Reche." *CatholicSaints.Info*. 8 April 2015. Web 25 December 2015.

10 - Saint Benedict of Nursia
- Benedict. "Chapter 36 – Of the Sick Brethren." *The Rule of St. Benedict.*
- "St. Benedict." *Butler's Lives of the Saints: New Full Edition:*
- *July*, Revised by Peter Doyle. Collegeville, MN: Burns & Oates/The Liturgical press, 1999, pp. 77-79.
- Contributors to Wikipedia. "Benedict of Nursia." *Wikipedia: The Free Encyclopedia*, 15 May 2017.

11 - Saint Benedict Menni
- "Bd. Benedict Menni." *Butler's Lives of the Saints: New Full Edition:*
- *April*, Revised by Peter Doyle. Collegeville, MN: Burns & Oates/The Liturgical press, 1999, pp. 177-179.
- "Benedict Menni (1841-1914)." *Vatican.va*, no date.
- Contributors to Wikipedia. "Benedict Menni." *Wikipedia: The Free Encyclopedia*, 20 October 2016.

12 - Blessed Benito Solana-Ruiz
- "Blessed Benito Solana-Ruiz." *CatholicSaints.Info*, no date.
- Contributors to Wikipedia. "Martyrs of Damiel." *Wikipedia: The Free Encyclopedia*, 12 April 2017.

13 - Blessed Bentivoglio de Bonis
- "Blessed Bentivoglio de Bonis." *CatholicSaints.Info*, 12 December 2009. Web 16 May 2017.
- "Bd. Bentivoglio de Bonis." *Butler's Lives of the Saints: New Full Edition:*
- *December*, Revised by Kathleen Jones. Collegeville, MN: Burns & Oates/The Liturgical press, 1999, pp. 196-197.

14 - Blessed Benvenuto of Gubbio
- "Bd. Benvenuto of Gubbio." *Butler's Lives of the Saints: New Full Edition: June*, Revised by Kathleen Jones. Collegeville, MN: Burns & Oates/The Liturgical press, 1999, pp. 212-213.
- "Bl. Benvenuto of Gubbio." *Catholic Online/Saints & Angels*, no date.

15 - Brother Bernadino of Obregón
- "Bernadino de Obregón: Un hombre de armas, un hombre de letras al Servicio de los pobres." *Biographia: Momentos de la Vida de Bernadino de Obregón: Causa de Beatificación y Canonización*, Portalhiades.com, 2009.
- Contributors to Wikipedia. "Obregonian Brothers." *Wikipedia: The Free Encyclopedia*, 15 August 2015.

16 - Saint Bernadino of Siena
- "St. Bernardino of Siena." *Butler's Lives of the Saints: New Full Edition:*
- *May*, Revised by David Hugh Farmer. Collegeville, MN: Burns & Oates/The Liturgical press, 1996, pp. 107-108.
- "St. Bernadine of Siena." *Catholic Online/Saints & Angels*, no date.
- Contributors to Wikipedia. "Bernadino of Siena." *Wikipedia: The Free Encyclopedia*, 19 December 2016.

17 - Saint Bernard of Corleone
- "Saint Bernard of Corleone." Capuchin Franciscan Friars of Australia, Province of the Assumption of Mary.
- "St. Bernard of Corleone." *CatholicCulture.org*, 2017.
- Contributors to Wikipedia. "Bernard of Corleone." *Wikipedia: The Free Encyclopedia*, 17 March 2017.

18 - Saint Bernardo Tolomei
- "Bd. Bernardo Tolomei." *Butler's Lives of the Saints: New Full Edition:*
- *August*, Revised by John Cumming. Collegeville, MN: Burns & Oates/The Liturgical press, 1998, pp. 203-204.
- Contributors to Wikipedia. "Bernardo Tolomei." *Wikipedia: The Free Encyclopedia*, 11 February 2017.
- "Bernardo Tolomei (1272-1348)." *Vatican.va*, no date.
- "St. Bernardo Tolomei." EWTN.

19 - Saint Cajetan
- Contributors to Wikipedia. "Saint Cajetan." *Wikipedia: The Free Encyclopedia*, 30 March 2017.

- "St. Cajetan." *Butler's Lives of the Saints: New Full Edition:*
- *August*, Revised by John Cumming. Collegeville, MN: Burns & Oates/The Liturgical press, 1998, pp. 46-48.
- "St. Cajetan." *Saint of the Day*, no date.

20 - Saint Camillus de Lellis
- Contributors to Wikipedia. "Camillus de Lellis." *Wikipedia: The Free Encyclopedia*, 6 May 2017.
- "St. Camillus de Lellis." *Butler's Lives of the Saints: New Full Edition:*
- *July*, Revised by Peter Doyle. Collegeville, MN: Burns & Oates/The Liturgical press, 1999, pp. 100-102.
- "St. Camillus de Lellis." *Catholic Online/Saints & Angels*, no date.
- "St. Camillus de Lellis." *Catholic Encyclopedia*. New York: Robert Appleton Company, 1908. Retrieved May 16, 2017, New Advent.

21 - Saint Carthach
- Contributors to Wikipedia. "Mo Chutu of Lismore." *Wikipedia: The Free Encyclopedia*, 13 May 2017.
- "St. Carthach." *Butler's Lives of the Saints: New Full Edition:*
- *May*, Revised by David Hugh Farmer. Collegeville, MN: Burns & Oates/The Liturgical press, 1996, pp. 77-78.

22 - Saint Charles of Sezze
- Contributors to Wikipedia. "Charles of Sezze." *Wikipedia: The Free Encyclopedia*, 30 March 2017.
- "St. Charles of Sezze." *Franciscan Media*, no date.
- "St. Charles of Sezze." *Catholic Online/Saints & Angels*, no date.
- "St. Charles of Sezze." *Stevenwoods.com*, no date.

23 - Saint Crispin of Viterbo
- "St. Crispin of Viterbo." *Butler's Lives of the Saints: New Full Edition: May*, Revised by David Hugh Farmer. Collegeville, MN: Burns & Oates/The Liturgical press, 1996, pp. 105-106.
- Contributors to Wikipedia. "Crispin of Viterbo." *Wikipedia: The Free Encyclopedia*, 30 November 2016.

- O'Neel, Brian. "The Ass of the Capuchins: Saint Crispin of Viterbo." Cincinnati, OH: Servant Books/St. Anthony Press, 2010, pp. 34-37.

24 - Saint Damien of Molokai
- "Bd. Damien De Veuster." *Butler's Lives of the Saints: New Full Edition:*
- *April*, Revised by Peter Doyle. Collegeville, MN: Burns & Oates/The Liturgical press, 1999, pp. 104-108.
- Matthew and Margaret Bunson. *Saint Damien of Molokai: Apostle to the Exiled.* Huntington, IN: Our Sunday Visitor Publications, 2009.
- Contributors to Wikipedia. "Father Damien." *Wikipedia: The Free Encyclopedia*, 25 June 2017.

25 - Saint Didacus (Diego)
- Contributors to Wikipedia. "Didacus of Alcalá." *Wikipedia: The Free Encyclopedia*, 31 October 2016.
- "St. Didacus." *Butler's Lives of the Saints: New Full Edition:*
- *November*, Revised by Sarah Fawcett Thomas. Collegeville, MN: Burns & Oates/The Liturgical Press, 1997, p. 110.
- "St. Didacus." *Saints & Angels: Catholic Online, no date.*

26 - Blessed Edward J.M. Poppe
- "Blessed Edward Poppe." *Catholic News Agency*, Friday, June 10, 2016.
- Contributors to Wikipedia. "Edward Poppe." *Wikipedia: The Free Encyclopedia*, 30 March 2017.
- Brian O'Neel. "Blessed Edward Poppe: In Love with the Eucharist." *39 New Saints You Should Know*. Cincinnati, OH: Servant Books, 2010, pp. 82-87.

27 - Blessed Engelmar Unzeitig
- "Fr. Engelmar Unzeitig." Trinity Stores, no date.
- "The Angel of Dachau: Pope Francis declares concentration camp priest a martyr." CNA/EWTN News, Jan. 26, 2016.

- "Fr. Engelmar Unzeitig, CMM (1911 – 1945). Marianhill Mission Society, no date.

28 - Blessed Enrico Rebuschini
- Brian O'Neel. "Blessed Enrico Rebuschini: Depression is Not the Final Word." *39 New Saints You Should Know.* Cincinnati, OH: Servant Books, 2010, pp. 109-112.
- "Bl. Enrico Rebuschini." *Catholic Online/Saints and Angels*, no date.
- Dom Antoine Marie. "Blessed Enrico Rebuschini Camillian. www.clairval.com 2002/11/25.

29 - Saint Fidelis of Sigmaringen
- Contributors to Wikipedia. "Fidelis of Sigmaringen." *Wikipedia: The Free Encyclopedia*, 31 January 2017.
- "St. Fidelis of Sigmaringen." *Butler's Lives of the Saints: New Full Edition:*
- *April,* Revised by Peter Doyle. Collegeville, MN: Burns & Oates/The Liturgical press, 1999, pp. 172-173.

30 - Saint Finnian of Clonard
- Contributors to Wikipedia. "Finnian of Clonard." *Wikipedia: The Free Encyclopedia*, 9 June 2017.
- "St. Finnian of Clonard." *Butler's Lives of the Saints: New Full Edition:*
- *December,* Revised by Kathleen Jones. Collegeville, MN: Burns & Oates/The Liturgical press, 1999, pp. 107-108.

31 - Saint Francis of Assisi
- Contributors to Wikipedia. "Francis of Assisi." *Wikipedia: The Free Encyclopedia*, 17 June 2017.
- "St. Francis of Assisi, Charismatic Penitent." The Franciscans, no date.
- "St. Francis of Assisi." *Butler's Lives of the Saints: New Full Edition:*
- *October,* Revised by Peter Doyle. Collegeville, MN: Burns & Oates/The Liturgical press, 1997, pp. 17-26.

32 - St. Francis Mary of Camporosso
- Contributors to Wikipedia. "Francesco Maria da Camporosso." *Wikipedia: The Free Encyclopedia*, 27 November 2016.
- "St. Francis Mary of Camporosso." *Butler's Lives of the Saints: New Full Edition: September,* Revised by Sarah Fawcett Thomas. Collegeville, MN: Burns & Oates/The Liturgical press, 1999, p. 171-172.
- "St. Francis Mary of Camporosso – A Man Can Have No Greater Love." Capuchin Saints. No date.

33 - St. Francis Xavier
- "St. Francis Xavier." *Butler's Lives of the Saints: New Full Edition: December,* Revised by Kathleen Jones. Collegeville, MN: Burns & Oates/The Liturgical press, 1999, pp. 25-30.
- "St. Francis Xavier." *Saint of the Day* for December 3.
- "St. Francis Xavier." *Catholic Online/Saints and Angels,* December 3.

34 - Blessed Francis Xavier Seelos
- Contributors to Wikipedia. "Francis Xavier Seelos." *Wikipedia: The Free Encyclopedia,* 19 June 2016.
- Rev. Carl Hoegerl. *The Life of Blessed Francis Xavier Seelos, Redemptorist,* Liguori, MO: Liguori, 2000.
- Fr. John Murray. "The Life of a Roving Redemptorist." Seelos.org.
- "Seelos Health Care." Seelos.org.

35 - Saint Gaspar Bertoni
- Contributors to Wikipedia. "Gaspare Bertoni." *Wikipedia: The Free Encyclopedia,* 12 August 2016.
- "Gaspar Bertoni (1777-1853): Priest, Founder of the Congregation of the Sacred Stigmata of Our Lord Jesus Christ." Biography, Vatican.va, no date.
- "St. Caspar Bertoni." *Butler's Lives of the Saints: New Full Edition:*
- *June,* Revised by Kathleen Jones. Collegeville, MN: Burns & Oates/The Liturgical press, 1997, pp. 99-100.

36 - Saint Gerard Majella
- Contributors to Wikipedia. "Gerard Majella." *Wikipedia: The Free Encyclopedia*, 24 June 2017.
- "Overview of the Life of St. Gerard Majella." Catholictradition.org. No date.
- "St. Gerard Majella." Catholic Online, no date.
- "St. Gerard Majella." *Butler's Lives of the Saints: New Full Edition:*
- *October,* Revised by Peter Doyle. Collegeville, MN: Burns & Oates/The Liturgical press, 1997, pp. 112-114.

37 - Blessed Gerard Meccati
- "Bd. Gerard Meccati." *Butler's Lives of the Saints: New Full Edition:*
- *May,* Revised by David Hugh Farmer. Collegeville, MN: Burns & Oates/The Liturgical press, 1996, pp. 72-73.
- Contributors to Wikipedia. "Gerard of Villamagna." *Wikipedia: The Free Encyclopedia*, 2 March 2017.

38 - Blessed Gerard Thom
- Contributors to Wikipedia. "Gerard Thom." *Wikipedia: The Free Encyclopedia*, no date.
- Contributors to Wikipedia. "Knights Hospitaller." *Wikipedia: The Free Encyclopedia*, 28 June 2017.

39 - Saint Gerlac
- Contributors to Wikipedia. "Saint Gerlac." *Wikipedia: The Free Encyclopedia*, 5 June 2017.
- "St. Gerlac." Norbertine Vocations Online, no date.
- "St. Gerlac." Catholic Online – Saints and Angels, no date.

40 - Saint Henry Morse
- Contributors to Wikipedia. "Henry Morse." *Wikipedia: The Free Encyclopedia*, 14 June 2017.
- "St. Henry Morse." *Butler's Lives of the Saints: New Full Edition:*
- *February,* Revised by Paul Burns. Collegeville, MN: Burns & Oates/The Liturgical press, 1998, pp. 9-10.

- "St. Henry Morse." St. Kateri Tekakwitha parish, Irondequoit, N.Y.
- "St. Henry Morse: Priest of the Plague." Mary's Downy Productions (DVD).

41 - Father Henri Nouwen
- Contributors to Wikipedia. "Henri Nouwen." *Wikipedia: The Free Encyclopedia*, 13 June 2017.
- Henri Nouwen. *Adam: God's Beloved*. Maryknoll, NY: Orbis Books, 1997.

42 - Blessed Hugolino Magalotti
- "Bd. Hugolino Magalotti." *Butler's Lives of the Saints: New Full Edition:*
- *December,* Revised by Kathleen Jones. Collegeville, MN: Burns & Oates/The Liturgical press, 1999, p. 99.
- "Beato Hugolino Magalotti: Ermitaño de la Tecera Orden." *Santoral Catholico Romano* Tracicional, no date.

43 - Saint Ivo of Brittany
- Contributors to Wikipedia. "Ivo of Kermartin." *Wikipedia: The Free Encyclopedia*, 8 June 2017.
- "St. Ivo of Brittany." *Butler's Lives of the Saints: New Full Edition:*
- *May,* Revised by David Hugh Farmer. Collegeville, MN: Burns & Oates/The Liturgical press, 1996, pp. 104-105.

44 - Blessed James of Bitetto
- "Bd. James of Bitetto." *Butler's Lives of the Saints: New Full Edition:*
- *April,* Revised by Peter Doyle. Collegeville, MN: Burns & Oates/The Liturgical press, 1999, pp. 193-194.
- "Blessed Jakov Varingez." Catholic Saints Info, no date.

45 - Blessed James of Lodi
- "Blessed James Oldo." CatholicSaints.Info. 18 April 2017.
- "Bd. James of Lodi." *Butler's Lives of the Saints: New Full Edition:*
- *April,* Revised by Peter Doyle. Collegeville, MN: Burns & Oates/The Liturgical press, 1999, p. 127.
- "Blessed James Oldo." Saint of the Day, no date.

46 - Blessed Jeremy of Valacchia

- "Blessed Geremia da Valacchia (1556-1652). From an article in Costanzo Cargnoni, *Sulle orme dei santi*, Rome, 2000, pp. 53-60.
- "Bd. Jeremy of Valacchia." *Butler's Lives of the Saints: New Full Edition:*
- *March,* Revised by Teresa Rodriguez. Collegeville, MN: Burns & Oates/The Liturgical press, 1999, pp. 47-48.
- Contributors to Wikipedia. "Jeremiah of Wallachia." *Wikipedia: The Free Encyclopedia*, 9 April 2017.

47 - Saint Jerome Emiliani

- Contributors to Wikipedia. "Gerolamo Emiliani." *Wikipedia: The Free Encyclopedia*, 8 June 2017.
- "St. Jerome Emiliani." *Butler's Lives of the Saints: New Full Edition:*
- *February,* Revised by Paul Burns. Collegeville, MN: Burns & Oates/The Liturgical press, 1998, pp. 78-79.
- "St. Jerome Emiliani." Catholic Online.

48 - Saint John Baptist Rossi

- Contributors to Wikipedia. "Giovanni Battista de' Rossi." *Wikipedia: The Free Encyclopedia*, 24 May 2017.
- "John Baptist Rossi." From *Saints Stories for All Ages*, Loyola University Press, online, no date.
- "St. John Baptist Rossi." *Butler's Lives of the Saints: New Full Edition:*
- *May,* Revised by David Hugh Farmer. Collegeville, MN: Burns & Oates/The Liturgical Press, 1996, p. 124.

49 - Saint John Bosco

- Contributors to Wikipedia. "John Bosco." *Wikipedia: The Free Encyclopedia*, 11 June 2017.
- "St. John Bosco." *Butler's Lives of the Saints: New Full Edition:*
- *January,* Revised by Paul Burns. Collegeville, MN: Burns & Oates/The Liturgical press, 1995, pp. 226-230.
- "St. John Bosco." *Catholic Encyclopedia*, 1913.

50 - St. John Calabria
- "Bd. John Calabria." *Butler's Lives of the Saints: New Full Edition:*
- *December,* Revised by Kathleen Jones. Collegeville, MN: Burns & Oates/The Liturgical press, 1999, p. 48.
- "John Calabria (1873-1954) - Priest, Founder of the Poor Servants and the Poor Women Servants of Divine Providence." Vatican.va Biography. No date.
- "St. Giovanni Calabria." Catholic Online – Saints and Angels, no date.

51 - Blessed John Colombini
- Contributors to Wikipedia. "Jesuati." *Wikipedia: The Free Encyclopedia*, 11 November 2016.
- "Bd. John Colombini." *Butler's Lives of the Saints: New Full Edition:*
- *July,* Revised by Peter Doyle. Collegeville, MN: Burns & Oates/The Liturgical press, 1999, pp. 261-262.

52 - Saint John of the Cross.
- Contributors to Wikipedia. "John of the Cross." *Wikipedia: The Free Encyclopedia*, 30 June 2017.
- "St. John of the Cross." *Butler's Lives of the Saints: New Full Edition:*
- *December,* Revised by Kathleen Jones. Collegeville, MN: Burns & Oates/The Liturgical press, 1999, pp. 121-127.

53 - Saint John Eudes
- Contributors to Wikipedia. "John Eudes." *Wikipedia: The Free Encyclopedia*, 8 June 2017.
- "St. John Eudes." *Butler's Lives of the Saints: New Full Edition:*
- *August,* Revised by John Cumming. Collegeville, MN: Burns & Oates/The Liturgical press, 1998, pp. 179-184.

54 - St. John of God
- Contributors to Wikipedia. "John of God." *Wikipedia: The Free Encyclopedia*, 23 March 2017.
- "St. John of God." *Butler's Lives of the Saints: New Full Edition:*

- *March,* Revised by Teresa Rodriguez. Collegeville, MN: Burns & Oates/The Liturgical press, 1999, pp. 69-74.
- "St. John of God." Catholic Online – Saints and Angels, no date.

55 - St. John Grande-Román
- Contributors to Wikipedia. "Juan Grande Román." *Wikipedia: The Free Encyclopedia*, 16 June 2017.
- "Bd. John 'The Sinner'." *Butler's Lives of the Saints: New Full Edition:*
- *June,* Revised by Kathleen Jones. Collegeville, MN: Burns & Oates/The Liturgical press, 1997, pp. 31-32.
- "St. Juan Grande Román." Vatican.va. Biography. No date.

56 - St. John Leonardi
- Contributors to Wikipedia. "Giovanni Leonardi." *Wikipedia: The Free Encyclopedia*, 30 March 2017.
- "St. John Leonardi." *Butler's Lives of the Saints: New Full Edition:*
- *October,* Revised by Peter Doyle. Collegeville, MN: Burns & Oates/The Liturgical press, 1997, pp. 52-53.

57 - Blessed John Pelingotto
- Contributors to Wikipedia. "Giovanni Pelingotto." *Wikipedia: The Free Encyclopedia*, 12 August 2016.
- "Bd. John Pelingotto." *Butler's Lives of the Saints: New Full Edition:*
- *June,* Revised by Kathleen Jones. Collegeville, MN: Burns & Oates/The Liturgical press, 1997, p. 20.
- "Blessed John Pelingotto." CatholicSaints.Info, 10 June 2017.

58 - Saint José Gabriel del Rosario Brochero
- "A Saint from Cordoba, Argentina." *Tipografia Vaticana*, no date.
- Contributors to Wikipedia. "José Gabriel del Rosario Brochero." *Wikipedia: The Free Encyclopedia*, 12 January 2017.
- Mary Rezac. "The Tale of Fr. Brochero: Gaucho Priest, Devil's Worst Nightmare." Catholic News Agency, December 28, 2016.
- Teresian Association. "Argentina: The 'Gaucho Priest,' José Gabriel del Rosario Brochero, Is Beatified." Published in *Spirituality/Evangelization*, no date.

59 - Blessed José Tarrats Comaposada
- "Beato José Tarrats Comaposada." *El Testigo Fiel*, 2013.
- "Blessed Josep Tarrats Comaposada." CatholicSaints.Info, 24 September 2015.
- "Blessed José Tarrats Comaposada." Jesuit Curia in Rome, 2017.

60 - Saint Joseph Cottolengo
- Contributors to Wikipedia. "Giuseppe Benedetto Cottolengo." *Wikipedia: The Free Encyclopedia*, 30 April 2017.
- "St. Joseph Cottolengo." *Butler's Lives of the Saints: New Full Edition:*
- *April*, Revised by Peter Doyle. Collegeville, MN: Burns & Oates/The Liturgical press, 1999, pp. 229-231.
- "St. Joseph Cottolengo." Saints and Angels – Catholic Online, no date.

61 - St. Joseph Calasanz
- Contributors to Wikipedia. "Joseph Calasanz." *Wikipedia: The Free Encyclopedia*, 10 May 2017.
- "St. Joseph Calasanz." *Butler's Lives of the Saints: New Full Edition:*
- *August*, Revised by John Cumming. Collegeville, MN: Burns & Oates/The Liturgical press, 1998, pp. 246-248.
- "St. Jos.eph Calasanz (1556-1648) Patron of Catholic Schools." CatholicIreland.net, no date.
- "St. Joseph Calasanz." Saint of the Day, no date.

62 - Brother Joseph Dutton
- Contributors to Wikipedia. "Joseph Dutton." *Wikipedia: The Free Encyclopedia*, 13 June 2017.
- Howard E. Couch. *Brother Dutton of Molokai*. Bellmore, NY: Damien-Dutton Society for Leprosy Aid, 2000.
- Olena Heu. "The Path to Sainthood: Brother Joseph Dutton." josephdutton@rcchawaii.org, April 10, 2014.
- Pat McNamara. "A Servant of the Lepers: Brother Joseph of Molokai." Catholic Education Resource Center, October 8, 2012.

63 - St. Joseph Freinademetz
- "Bd. Joseph Freinademetz." *Butler's Lives of the Saints: New Full Edition:*
- *January,* Revised by Paul Burns. Collegeville, MN: Burns & Oates/The Liturgical press, 1995, pp. 214-217.
- Contributors to Wikipedia. "Joseph Freinademetz." *Wikipedia: The Free Encyclopedia*, 30 June 2017.
- "Joseph Freinademetz (1852-1908)." Vatican.va Biography, no date.

64 - Blessed Joseph Gerard
- Contributors to Wikipedia. "Joseph Gérard." *Wikipedia: The Free Encyclopedia*, 11 May 2017.
- "Bd. Joseph Gerard." *Butler's Lives of the Saints: New Full Edition:*
- *May,* Revised by David Hugh Farmer. Collegeville, MN: Burns & Oates/The Liturgical press, 1996, p. 166.
- "Blessed Joseph Gérard Missionary of Lesotho." OMI Postulation. ENG, no date.

65 - Saint Joseph Oriol
- Contributors to Wikipedia. "Joseph Oriol." *Wikipedia: The Free Encyclopedia*, 24 September 2016.
- "St. Joseph Oriol." *Butler's Lives of the Saints: New Full Edition:*
- *March,* Revised by Teresa Rodriguez. Collegeville, MN: Burns & Oates/The Liturgical press, 1999, p. 230-232.
- "St. Joseph Oriol: Apostle of Barcelona." Iconographie Chrétienne, 23 March 2015 (several articles in various languages).

66 - Blessed Juan Augustín Codera-Marqués
- "Blessed Juan Augustín Codera-Marqués." CatholicSaints.Info, 21 September 2015.
- "Blessed Juan Augustín Codera-Marqués." CatholicSaints.Info, 29 July 2016.

67 - Blessed Juan Bautista Egozcuezábal-Aldaz
- "Blessed Juan Bautista Egozcuezábal-Aldaz." CatholicSaints.Info 29 July 2015.

- "Blessed Juan Bautista Egozcuezábal-Aldaz." CatholicSaints.Info Saints Who Were Nurses, 29 July 2016.

68 - Saint Juan Macías
- Contributors to Wikipedia. "John Macias." *Wikipedia: The Free Encyclopedia*, 25 April 2017.
- "St. John Macías." *Butler's Lives of the Saints: New Full Edition:*
- *September,* Revised by Sarah Fawcett Thomas. Collegeville, MN: Burns & Oates/The Liturgical press, 1999, p. 154.

69 - Brother Juan de Mena
- Chad O'Lynn. *Men in Nursing: History, Challenges, and Opportunities.* New York, NY: Springer Publishing Company, 2006.
- Thunderwolf. "Friar Juan de Mena." Allnurses, 25 August 2015.
- Robert S. Weddle. "Mena, Marcos de." *Handbook of Texas Online*, June 15, 2010.

70 - St. Justin de Jacobis
- Contributors to Wikipedia. "Giustino de Jacobis." *Wikipedia: The Free Encyclopedia*, 24 February 2017.
- Famvin. "Justin de Jacobis." *Vincentian Encyclopedia*, no date.
- "St. Justin de Jacobis." *Butler's Lives of the Saints: New Full Edition:*
- *July,* Revised by Peter Doyle. Collegeville, MN: Burns & Oates/The Liturgical press, 1999, p. 263-265.
- "St. Justin de Jacobis, Evangelist in Ethiopia." Agenzia Fides. July 30, 2011.

71 - Blessed Liberatus Weiss
- ""BB Liberatus Weiss, Samuel Marzorati, and Michael Fasoli." *Butler's Lives of the Saints: New Full Edition: March,* Revised by Teresa Rodriguez. Collegeville, MN: Burns & Oates/The Liturgical press, 1999, pp. 29-31.

72 - Blessed Luchesio Modestini
- Contributors to Wikipedia. "Luchesius Modestini." *Wikipedia: The Free Encyclopedia*, 6 July 2016.

- "Bd. Luchesio." *Butler's Lives of the Saints: New Full Edition: April,* Revised by Peter Doyle. Collegeville, MN: Burns & Oates/ The Liturgical press, 1999, pp. 198-199.
- "St. Luchesio." Saints and Angels, no date.

73 - St. Louis Bertrán
- Contributors to Wikipedia. "Louis Bertrand." *Wikipedia: The Free Encyclopedia*, 20 December 2016.
- "St. Louis Bertrán." *Butler's Lives of the Saints: New Full Edition: October,* Revised by Peter Doyle. Collegeville, MN: Burns & Oates/The Liturgical press, 1997, pp. 57-58
- "St. Louis Bertrand." CatholicSaints.Info, 10 October 2016.

74 - Saint Ludovico of Casoria
- Contributors to Wikipedia. "Ludovico of Casoria." *Wikipedia: The Free Encyclopedia*, 16 October 2016.
- EWTN. "St. Ludovico da Casoria." Canonizations 1993-2016.
- "Saint Ludovico of Casoria." Franciscan Media, no date.

75 - Blessed Luigi Maria Monti
- "Blessed Luigi Maria Monti." CatholicSaints.Info, 19 May 2016.
- "Blessed Luigi Maria Monti." CatholicSaints.Info – Saints Who Were Nurses, 21 October 2008.
- "Founder." CFIC North American Delegation, 2012.

76 - Blessed Luke Belluti
- "Bd. Luke Belluti." *Butler's Lives of the Saints: New Full Edition: February,* Revised by Paul Burns. Collegeville, MN: Burns & Oates/The Liturgical press, 1998, pp. 173-174.
- "Blessed Luke Belluti." Saint of the Day Franciscan Media, no date.

77 - Saint Martin de Porres
- Contributors to Wikipedia. "Martin de Porres." *Wikipedia: The Free Encyclopedia*, 24 June 2017.
- "St. Martin de Porres." *Butler's Lives of the Saints: New Full Edition: November,* Revised by Sarah Fawcett Thomas. Collegeville, MN: Burns & Oates/The Liturgical press, 1997, pp. 18-20.
- "St. Martin de Porres." Saint of the Day, no date.

78 - Blessed Michael Pius Fasoli
- [Please see Blessed Liberatus Weiss]
- "Blessed Michele Pío Fasoli." CatholicSaints.Info, 6 September 2016.

79 - Saint Michael Kozaki
- "Saint Michael Kozaki." CatholicSaints.Info, 13 August 2016.
- "Saint Michael Kozaki." CatholicSaints.Info, "Saints Who Were Nurses," 21 October 2008.
- "St. Michael Kozaki." Saints and Angels, no date.

80 - Blessed Michael Rua
- Contributors to Wikipedia. "Michele Rua." *Wikipedia: The Free Encyclopedia*, 28 December 2016.
- "Bd. Michael Rua." *Butler's Lives of the Saints: New Full Edition:*
- *April,* Revised by Peter Doyle. Collegeville, MN: Burns & Oates/The Liturgical press, 1999, pp. 40-42.

81 - Venerable Nicola D'Onofrio
- Contributors to Wikipedia. "Nicola D'Onofrio." *Wikipedia: The Free Encyclopedia*, 15 December 2016.
- "Servant of God Nicola D'Onofrio." Order of St. Camillus – Ministers of the Sick, 2015.
- "Venerable Nicola D'Onofrio." CatholicSaints.Info, 30 October 2016.

82 - Blessed Oddino Barrotti
- Marion A. Habig. "Blessed Oddino Barrotti." *The Franciscan Book of Saints, no date.*
- "Bd. Oddino of Fossano." *Butler's Lives of the Saints: New Full Edition:*
- *June,* Revised by Kathleen Jones. Collegeville, MN: Burns & Oates/The Liturgical press, 1997, pp. 51-52.
- "Blessed Oddino Barrotti." CatholicSaints.Info, 7 July 2016.

83 - Saint Paul of the Cross
- Contributors to Wikipedia. "Paul of the Cross." *Wikipedia: The Free Encyclopedia*, 20 October 2016.

- "St. Paul of the Cross." *Butler's Lives of the Saints: New Full Edition:*
- *October,* Revised by Peter Doyle. Collegeville, MN: Burns & Oates/The Liturgical press, 1997, pp. 130-133.

84 - Saint Peter of St. Joseph de Betancur
- Contributors to Wikipedia. "Peter of Saint Joseph de Betancur." *Wikipedia: The Free Encyclopedia*, 22 November 2016.
- "Bd. Peter de Betancur." *Butler's Lives of the Saints: New Full Edition:*
- *June,* Revised by Kathleen Jones. Collegeville, MN: Burns & Oates/The Liturgical press, 1997, p. 186.
- "St. Peter de Betancurt (1626-1667). Vatican.va Biography, no date.

85 - St. Peter Claver
- Contributors to Wikipedia. "Peter Claver." *Wikipedia: The Free Encyclopedia*, 25 June 2017.
- "St. Peter Claver." *Butler's Lives of the Saints: New Full Edition:*
- *June,* Revised by Kathleen Jones. Collegeville, MN: Burns & Oates/The Liturgical press, 1997, pp. 76-80.
- "St. Peter Claver." Knights of St. Peter Claver, no date.

86 - Blessed Peter Donders
- Contributors to Wikipedia. "Peter Donders." *Wikipedia: The Free Encyclopedia*, 24 March 2017.
- "Bd. Peter Donders." *Butler's Lives of the Saints: New Full Edition:*
- *January,* Revised by Paul Burns. Collegeville, MN: Burns & Oates/The Liturgical press, 1995, pp. 102-103.
- "Blessed Peter Donders." The Redemptorists, no date.

87 - Blessed Peter Tecelano
- Contributors to Wikipedia. "Peter Tecelano." *Wikipedia: The Free Encyclopedia*, 19 December 2016.
- "Blessed Peter Tecelano." Catholic Online, no date.
- "Blessed Peter Tecelano." CatholicSaints.Info, 30 June 2016.
- "Bd. Peter of Siena." *Butler's Lives of the Saints: New Full Edition:*

- *December*, Revised by Kathleen Jones. Collegeville, MN: Burns & Oates/The Liturgical press, 1999, pp. 45-46.

88 - Saint Philip Neri
- Contributors to Wikipedia. "Philip Neri." *Wikipedia: The Free Encyclopedia*, 24 June 2017.
- "St. Philip Neri." *Butler's Lives of the Saints: New Full Edition: May*, Revised by David Hugh Farmer. Collegeville, MN: Burns & Oates/The Liturgical press, 1996, pp. 144-147.

89 - Blessed Pier Giorgio Frassati
- Maria Di Lorenzo. *Blessed Pier Giorgio Frassati: An Ordinary Christian*. Boston: Pauline Books and Media, 2004.
- "Bl. Pier Giorgio Frassati." Catholic Online – Saints and Angels, no date.
- Contributors to Wikipedia. "Pier Giorgio Frassati." *Wikipedia: The Free Encyclopedia*, 27 June 2017.
- Cristina Siccardi. *Pier Giorgio Frassati: A Hero for Our Times*. San Francisco: Ignatius Press, 2016.

90 - Blessed Raphael Chylinski
- "Bd. Raphael Chylinsky." *Butler's Lives of the Saints: New Full Edition:*
- *December*, Revised by Kathleen Jones. Collegeville, MN: Burns & Oates/The Liturgical press, 1999, pp. 23-24.
- "Bl. Rafael Chylinski." Catholic Online/Saints & Angels, no date.
- "Blessed Rafal Chylinski." Saint of the Day, no date.

91 - Blessed Raymond of Capua
- Contributors to Wikipedia. "Raymond of Capua." *Wikipedia: The Free Encyclopedia*, 5 November 2016.
- "Bd. Raymond of Capua." *Butler's Lives of the Saints: New Full Edition:*
- *October*, Revised by Peter Doyle. Collegeville, MN: Burns & Oates/The Liturgical press, 1997, pp. 31-33.
- Dorcy, Sr. Marie Jean. "Blessed Raymond of Capua." *St. Dominic's Family*. Tan Books and Publishers, 1983.

Selected Bibliography

92 - St. Rock
- Contributors to Wikipedia. "Saint Roch." *Wikipedia: The Free Encyclopedia*, 24 June 2017.
- "St. Rock." *Butler's Lives of the Saints: New Full Edition: August*, Revised by John Cumming. Collegeville, MN: Burns & Oates/The Liturgical press, 1998, pp. 162-164.
- "St. Roch." Catholic Online/Saints & Angels, no date.

93 - Saint Salvius of Albi
- "St. Salvius of Albi." *Butler's Lives of the Saints: New Full Edition:*
- *September,* Revised by Sarah Fawcett Thomas. Collegeville, MN: Burns & Oates/The Liturgical press, 1999, pp. 89-90.
- "St. Salvius of Albi." Saints & Angels, no date.

94 - Blessed Samuel Marzorati
- [Please see St. Liberatus Weiss.]
- "Blessed Antonio Francesco Marzorati." CatholicSaints.Info, 28 February 2017.

95 - Saint Simon of Lipnicza
- Contributors to Wikipedia. "Szymon of Lipnica." *Wikipedia: The Free Encyclopedia*, 6 May 2017.
- "Bd. Simon of Lipnicza." *Butler's Lives of the Saints: New Full Edition:*
- *July,* Revised by Peter Doyle. Collegeville, MN: Burns & Oates/The Liturgical press, 1999, pp. 146-147.
- "Blessed Simon of Lipnica (1435-1440). Vatican.va Biography, no date.

96 - Venerable Simon Srugi
- Ernesto Forti, translated by Fr. Prospero Roero, SDB. *Venerable Simon Srugi: Salesian of Nazareth*, no date.
- "Ven. Simon Srugi." Salesian Missions Online, no date.

97 - Blessed Stephen Bellesini
- Contributors to Wikipedia. "Stephen Bellesini." *Wikipedia: The Free Encyclopedia*, 29 April 2016.
- "Bd. Stephen Bellesini." *Butler's Lives of the Saints: New Full Edition:*

- *February*, Revised by Paul Burns. Collegeville, MN: Burns & Oates/The Liturgical press, 1998, p. 21.
- Gary N. McCloskey, OSA. "Blessed Stephen Bellesini." St. Thomas of Villanova Monastery, Villanova, Pennsylvania, no date.

98 - St. Toribio Romo-González
- Contributors to Wikipedia. "Toribio Romo González." *Wikipedia: The Free Encyclopedia*, 24 February 2017.
- Alfredo Corchado. "The Migrant's Saint: Toribio Romo." *The Dallas Morning News*, Saturday, July 22, 2016.
- Fr. Robert J. Kus. "San Toribio Romo González: El Santo Coyote," Rincón del Espíritu, *La Prensa de las Carolinas*, October 2018, p. 18.
- Bob Lord and Penny Lord. "Saint Toribio Romo: Patron of Immigrants." No date.

99 - Blessed Vivaldi Stricchi
- Kevin Elphick. "Bartolo and Vivaldo." Jesus in Love Blog, 10 December 2014.
- Fr. Don Miller, OFM. "Blessed Waldo." Franciscan Media: Saint of the Day, no date.
- "Who Was Vivaldi Stricchi?" The Holy Mount, San Vivaldo, Montaione, Tuscany, Italy, no date.

100 - Saint Zygmunt Gorazdowski
- Contributors to Wikipedia. "Zygmunt Gorazdowski." *Wikipedia: The Free Encyclopedia*, 24 May 2017.
- "Zygmunt Gorazdowski (1845-1920) Priest, Founder of the Congregation of the Sisters of St. Joseph." ETWN, no date.
- "St. Zygmunt Gorazdowski." Catholic Online/Saints & Angels, no date.

www.ingramcontent.com/pod-product-compliance
Lightning Source LLC
Chambersburg PA
CBHW020733180526
45163CB00001B/222